Interventional Radiology Cases

Published and forthcoming books in the *Cases in Radiology* series:

Body MRI Cases, William Brant and Eduard de Lange

Breast Imaging Cases, Catherine Appleton and Kimberly Wiele

Cardiac Imaging Cases, Charles White and Joseph Jen-Sho Chen

Chest Imaging Cases, Sanjeev Bhalla, Cylen Javidan-Nejad, Kristopher W. Cummings, and Andrew Bierhals

Emergency Radiology Cases, Hani Abujudeh

Gastrointestinal Imaging Cases, Angela Levy, Koenraad Mortele, and Benjamin Yeh

Genitourinary Imaging Cases, Mark Lockhart and Rupan Sanyal

Interventional Radiology Cases, Anne M. Covey, Bradley B. Pua, Allison Aguado, and David C. Madoff

Musculoskeletal Imaging Cases, Mark Anderson and Stacy Smith

Neuroradiology Cases, Clifford Eskey, Clifford Belden, David Pastel, Arastoo Vossough, and Albert Yoo

Nuclear Medicine Cases, Chun Kim

Pediatric Imaging Cases, Ellen Chung

Ultrasound Cases, Leslie Scoutt, Ulrike Hamper, and Teresita Angtuaco

Interventional Radiology Cases

Anne M. Covey, MD

Associate Professor of Radiology
Memorial Sloan-Kettering Cancer Center
Weill Cornell Medical College
New York, New York

Bradley B. Pua, MD

Assistant Professor of Radiology
Weill Cornell Medical College
New York Presbyterian Hospital
New York, New York

Allison Aguado, MD

Assistant Professor of Radiology
Memorial Sloan-Kettering Cancer Center
Weill Cornell Medical College
New York, New York

David C. Madoff, MD

Chief of Interventional Radiology
Professor of Radiology
Weill Cornell Medical College
New York Presbyterian Hospital
New York, New York

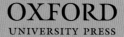

OXFORD
UNIVERSITY PRESS

OXFORD
UNIVERSITY PRESS

Oxford University Press is a department of the University of Oxford.
It furthers the University's objective of excellence in research, scholarship,
and education by publishing worldwide.

Oxford   New York
Auckland   Cape Town   Dar es Salaam   Hong Kong   Karachi
Kuala Lumpur   Madrid   Melbourne   Mexico City   Nairobi
New Delhi   Shanghai   Taipei   Toronto

With offices in
Argentina   Austria   Brazil   Chile   Czech Republic   France   Greece
Guatemala   Hungary   Italy   Japan   Poland   Portugal   Singapore
South Korea   Switzerland   Thailand   Turkey   Ukraine   Vietnam

Oxford is a registered trademark of Oxford University Press
in the UK and certain other countries.

Published in the United States of America by
Oxford University Press
198 Madison Avenue, New York, NY 10016

Library of Congress Cataloging-in-Publication Data
Covey, Anne M., author.
Interventional radiology cases / Anne M. Covey, Bradley B. Pua, Allison Aguado, David C. Madoff.
p. ; cm.—(Cases in radiology)
Includes bibliographical references and indexes.
ISBN 978-0-19-933127-7 (alk. paper)
I. Pua, Bradley B., author.   II. Aguado, Allison, author.   III. Madoff, David C., author.   IV. Title.
V. Series: Cases in radiology.
[DNLM: 1. Radiology, Interventional—methods—Case Reports. WN 180]
RC78
616.07'57—dc23   2014005736

This material is not intended to be, and should not be considered, a substitute for medical or other
professional advice. Treatment for the conditions described in this material is highly dependent on
the individual circumstances. And, while this material is designed to offer accurate information with
respect to the subject matter covered and to be current as of the time it was written, research and
knowledge about medical and health issues is constantly evolving and dose schedules for medications
are being revised continually, with new side effects recognized and accounted for regularly. Readers
must therefore always check the product information and clinical procedures with the most up-to-date
published product information and data sheets provided by the manufacturers and the most recent
codes of conduct and safety regulation. The publisher and the authors make no representations or
warranties to readers, express or implied, as to the accuracy or completeness of this material. Without
limiting the foregoing, the publisher and the authors make no representations or warranties as to the
accuracy or efficacy of the drug dosages mentioned in the material. The authors and the publisher do
not accept, and expressly disclaim, any responsibility for any liability, loss, or risk that may be claimed
or incurred as a consequence of the use and/or application of any of the contents of this material.

9 8 7 6 5 4 3 2 1
Printed in China

To my incredible daughters, Emma and Olivia (Rainy), who mean the world to me

—*Anne M. Covey*

To my parents, wife, and sister for their continued love and support

—*Bradley B. Pua*

Special thanks to my wife Esa, and my children Emma, Benjamin and Samuel for whom without their support, this work would not have been possible.

—*David C. Madoff*

Acknowledgments

The publisher thanks the following for their time and advice:

Mark Anderson, University of Virginia

Sanjeev Bhalla, Mallinckrodt Institute of Radiology, Washington University

Michael Bruno, Penn State Hershey Medical Center

Melissa Rosado de Christenson, St. Luke's Hospital of Kansas City

Rihan Khan, University of ArizonaAngela Levy, Georgetown University

Alexander Mamourian, University of Pennsylvania

Stacy Smith, Brigham and Women's Hospital

Case 62: Images courtesy of Neil M. Khilnani, MD, Weill Cornell Medical College, New York, NY

Case 64: Images courtesy of Rotimi O. Johnson, MD, St. Louis University School of Medicine, St Louis, MO

Case 77: Images courtesy of George G. Vatakencherry, MD, Kaiser Permanente Medical Group, Rancho Cucamonga, CA

Cases 47 and 103: Case submitted by Bedros Taslakian, MD, American University of Beirut Medical Center, Beirut, Lebanon

Preface

The world of interventional radiology is changing. Over the next several years we will transition to a residency in interventional radiology to provide a more clinically based experience for trainees with time dedicated to critical care, surgery, and medicine. And over the past decade, the focus of many practices has shifted from peripheral vascular intervention to interventional oncology. One thing that has not changed, however, is the importance of case review and self-assessment in developing the breadth and depth of knowledge required to become a skilled interventional radiologist.

We are absolutely amazed when we look over the impressive CVs of fellow and junior attending applicants. If being a good doctor could simply be achieved by dedication, research, and community service, they would all be outstanding at the start. But the fact is that experience counts—and as it turns out, it counts for quite a lot.

Experience can be gained in many ways. Being directly involved in the workup, case, and follow-up management is the best way to learn. Doing cases alone, however, is not enough. Knowledge can be supplemented with lectures, conferences, and ongoing review of cases, and particularly unknown cases. This book is written with that in mind. The cases that follow are presented as unknowns, some with direct questions posed to the reader and many without. It is our intention that this book will be used in different ways by readers at different levels.

The structure of each case—images and short clinical history on one page and detailed annotated images, teaching points, and management outlined on the following page(s)—allows it to be used by residents early in their training, and they will benefit by using it as a complement to a more thorough text and as a quick reference for upcoming cases. More advanced residents and fellows will use it as an opportunity for self-assessment and to supplement their knowledge. Practicing radiologists can keep it handy to use as a quick refresher for cases they do infrequently, such as adrenal vein sampling.

Of course, the experience of studying these cases is not intended to substitute for hands-on experience. Unlike other casebooks, the focus is on radiographic findings and diagnosis; we have key teaching points and management issues that are so critical in taking good care of patients. Interventional radiologists today are active clinicians, no longer proceduralists, with many seeing patients in clinic and with hospital admitting privileges. In years past, questions once posed to referring doctors, such as "When can my abscess catheter be removed?" and

"When should I be reimaged after treatment of my liver tumor?" are being asked directly to the interventional radiologist. These are some of the important management issues we have included for the reader.

In training scores of residents and fellows, we have shared many tips that we have found helpful in our ongoing education. An important one is to challenge someone taking a case to synthesize the case out loud. When we show cases to a group of residents or fellows and ask a question to the person in the proverbial hot seat, invariably there are self-congratulatory nods from several members of the audience before the person taking the case has finished reviewing the images. When the answer is revealed, they pat themselves on the back because they "would have said that." Only when readers verbalize their findings and syntheses of cases can they really know what they "would have said" because they would have said it.

The references were carefully chosen to be clinically relevant, and they are here to provide additional resources, many generally accepted as white papers or standards that provide for more in-depth reading.

Finally, but not lastly, we would like to thank Andrea Seils, who proposed this project to us several years ago and waited patiently, providing all of the guidance and resources we needed to make it happen. This book never would have happened without the support and encouragement of Andrea and her fantastic team at Oxford University Press.

Contents

Venous Access:

Cases 1–6   1–18

Biopsy:

Cases 7–20   19–59

Ablation:

Cases 21–26   60–77

Embolization:

Cases 27–45   78–134

Genitourinary Intervention:

Cases 46–51   135–152

Gastrointestinal/Biliary Intervention:

Cases 52–61   153–181

Venous Intervention:

Cases 62–75   182–229

Arterial Intervention:

Cases 76–85   230–259

Case 86   260–262

Cases 87–92   263–279

Drainage:

Cases 93–101   280–304

Spine Augmentation:

Case 102   305–307

Case 103   308–312

History

▶ Colon Cancer (Needs Vascular Access for Chemotherapy)

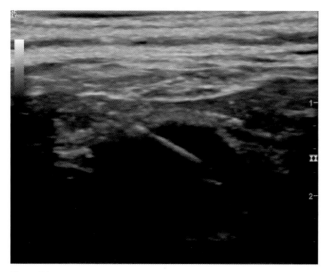

Figure 1.1

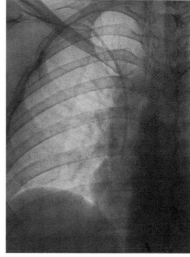

Figure 1.2

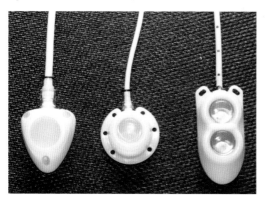

Figure 1.3

Case 1 Mediport

Figure 1.4

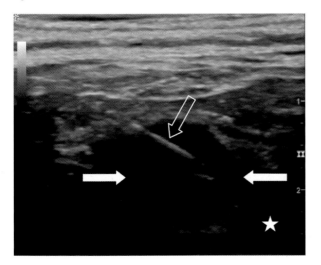

Figure 1.5

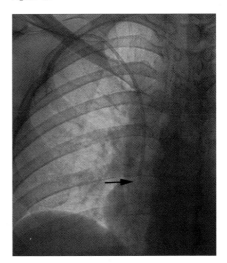

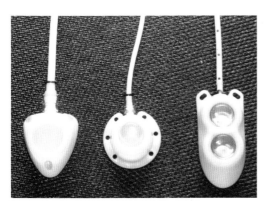

Figure 1.6

Findings

▸ Ultrasound shows the internal jugular vein to be patent (arrows) in its typical location lateral to the carotid artery (Fig. 1.4, star). The needle (hollow arrow) is entering the vein from a lateral approach above the clavicle.

▸ Spot fluoroscopic image shows the implantable venous access device (IVAD) over the right chest wall attached to the catheter entering the internal jugular vein and terminating at the expected location of the cavoatrial junction (Fig. 1.5, arrow).

▸ Figure 1.6 shows some of the different configurations of available devices. From the left is a Bard Power Port, which supports a flow rate of up to 5 cc/second. In the middle is a standard single-lumen port with tissue ingrowth holes that can also be used for retention sutures. On the right is a dual-lumen device. Note it is attached to a single catheter that has a septum separating the two lumens.

Teaching Points

▸ IVADs are good catheters for long-term, intermittent use making them ideal for administration of intravenous chemotherapy.

- Internal jugular vein is preferred to subclavian vein access for several reasons. With ultrasound-guided internal jugular access, there is almost no risk of pneumothorax. Pericatheter thrombus in the internal jugular vein is most often asymptomatic whereas in the subclavian vein it can cause significant morbidity in the form of upper-extremity swelling. Even asymptomatic catheter-related stenosis in the subclavian vein may prevent use of the extremity for dialysis graft/fistula maturation in the future. Finally, subclavian vein catheters are subject to the possibility of "pinch-off syndrome" in which repetitive motion of the upper extremity is complicated by catheter fracture (see Case 4).
- Ideal catheter tip location is the cavoatrial junction or high right atrium. Catheters left higher in the superior vena cava are prone to cause strictures, fibrin sheath, and thrombus. While the exact location of the cavoatrial junction is impossible to predict with fluoroscopy, it is approximated in children at two vertebral bodies below the carina, and in adults approximately 4 cm below the carina.

Management

- IVADs may be left in place as long as they are needed. Most manufacturers recommend that the catheters should be flushed regularly at 4-week intervals with saline (valved catheters) or heparinized saline.
- IVAD placement is a clean procedure, and the use of prophylactic antibiotics has not been shown to prevent placement-related infection. Procedure-related infections (i.e., within 30 days of placement) are seen in approximately 1%–2% of cases.
- Safe access to puncture the silicone septum of the resevoir is achieved with a Huber needle, which is a noncoring, long-bevel, hollow needle.

Further Reading

Gonda SJ, Li R. Principles of subcutaneous port placement. *Tech Vasc Interv Radiol*. 2011; 14(4):198–203.
Walser EM. Venous access ports: indications, implantation technique, follow-up, and complications. *Cardiovasc Intervent Radiol*. 2012; 35(4):751–764.

History

► Lung Cancer and Superior Vena Cava Occlusion; Requires Access for Chemotherapy. What procedure is being performed?

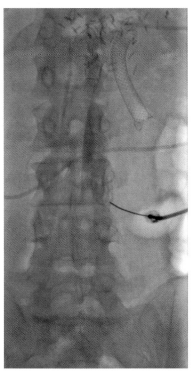

Figure 2.1

Case 2   Translumbar Placement of Implantable Venous Access Device

Figure 2.2

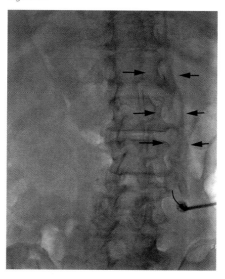

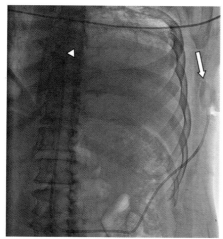

Figure 2.3

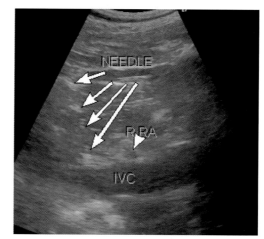

Figure 2.4

Findings

▶ A needle is seen overlying the third lumbar vertebra (Fig. 2.2). Contrast injection opacifies the inferior vena cava (IVC; arrows).

▶ A translumbar implantable venous access device (IVAD) has been placed (Fig. 2.3) entering the IVC at the L3 vertebral level with the catheter terminating at the expected location of the cavo-atrial junction (arrowhead). The port resevoir is seen over the lateral lower chest wall (arrow).

▶ In another patient, ultrasound guidance was used for IVC access and to identify (and avoid) the right renal artery (Fig. 2.4).

Teaching Points

▶ In patients who need central venous access and have superior vena cava occlusion or occlusion of internal jugular, external jugular, and subclavian veins, translumbar access may be performed. Alternative access sites include femoral, hepatic, and renal veins in patients with renal failure.

▶ Access to the IVC may be achieved with fluoroscopic guidance or ultrasound guidance in thin patients; occasionally computed tomography (CT) guidance may be required. To minimize the risk of injury to the renal vasculature, access should be below the L2-L3 interspace.

▶ Using fluoroscopic guidance, the anterolateral vertebral body can be used for reference, and the needle can be "walked off" the lateral aspect of the vertebra and directed anteriorly and medially to the expected location of the inferior vena cava. Aspiration of blood from the needle confirms intravascular location, and contrast can be injected to confirm position within the cava (Fig. 2.1).

Management

▶ Translumbar IVADs can be used in the same manner as devices placed on the chest wall or upper extremity. The length of the catheter needed is longer, often 70 cm, and the 65 cm catheters that are packaged with some IVADs may be too short.

▶ Catheters should be flushed with sterile saline or heparin every 4 weeks to minimize the risk of catheter occlusion and formation of biofilm within the lumen of the catheter.

▶ The device should be placed over the lower lateral/anterorlateral chest wall to facilitate access. If the port is placed in the soft tissue of the abdomen without the buttress of the rib cage, it may be very difficult to access.

Further Reading

Denny DF Jr. Venous access salvage techniques. *Tech Vasc Interv Radiol.* 2011; 14(4):225–232.

History

► A 9-Month-Old Boy with Congenital Heart Disease for Peripherally Inserted Central Catheter Placement
  Where is the Tip of the Left Sided Catheter?

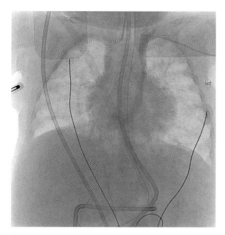

Figure 3.1

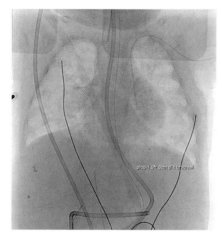

Figure 3.2

Case 3   Left Superior Vena Cava

Figure 3.3

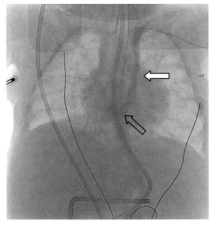

Figure 3.4

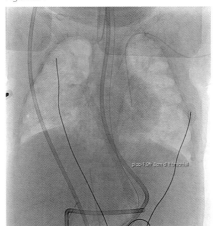

Figure 3.5

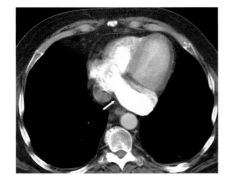

Figure 3.6

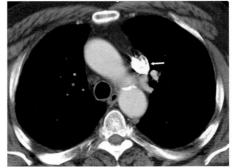

Figure 3.7

Findings

▶ Venogram during placement of left-sided central line (Fig. 3.3) demonstrates a persistent left-sided superior vena cava (SVC; arrow) draining into the coronary sinus (hollow arrow).

▶ After placement of the central line, the catheter is seen to the left of the spine within the left-sided SVC (Fig. 3.4).

▶ Contrast enhanced CT of another patient demonstrates a left-sided SVC (Fig. 3.6, arrow) draining into the coronary sinus (Fig. 3.5, arrow) at the posterior aspect of the right atrium. Note the absence of the right-sided SVC in its expected location to the right of the aortic arch.

▶ Venogram from a different patient (Fig. 3.7) shows a catheter placed via the left internal jugular vein (arrow) communicating with a branch of the left pulmonary vein (hollow arrow). This anomaly was also discovered at the time of central line placement.

Teaching Points

▶ The most common anomaly of the SVC is duplication. Persistent left SVC with absence of a right SVC is uncommon, seen in <1% of the general population and in 4%–11% of patients with congenital heart disease.

▶ Persistent left SVC is due to failure of regression of the left anterior, common cardinal veins, and left sinus horn.

▶ Left SVC most often drains into an enlarged coronary sinus.
Rarely a persistent left SVC drains directly into the left atrium and as a right-to-left shunt can be a source of paradoxical emboli.

▶ Partial anomalous pulmonary venous return occurs when a pulmonary vein communicates with the right atrium or a systemic vein (as in Fig. 3.7), resulting in a left-to-right shunt.

Management

▶ In addition to persistent left SVC, the differential for abnormal course of a wire or catheter during line placement should include intra-arterial placement and partial anomalous pulmonary venous return.

▶ Careful attention to prior imaging, when available, can alert the astute operator to venous anomalies.

Further Reading

Burney K, Young H, Barnard SA, McCoubrie P, Darby M. CT appearances of congenital and acquired abnormalities of the superior vena cava. *Clin Radiol.* 2007;62(9):837–842.

Fares WH, Birchard KR, Yankaskas JR. Persistent left superior vena cava identified during central line placement: a case report. *Respir Med CME.* 2011; 4(3):141–143.

{

History

▶ Pain on Injection of Implantable Venous Access Device

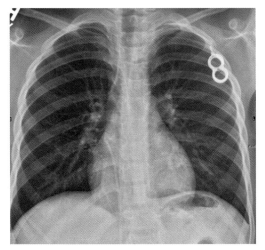

Figure 4.1

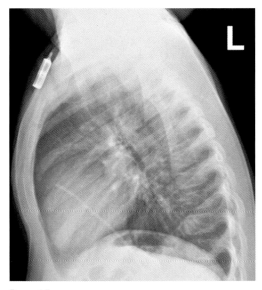

Figure 4.2

Case 4   Port Catheter Dislodged from Reservoir

Figure 4.3

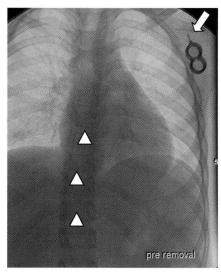

Figure 4.4

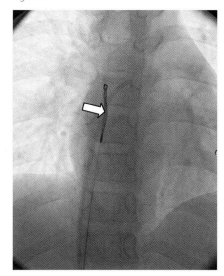

Figure 4.5

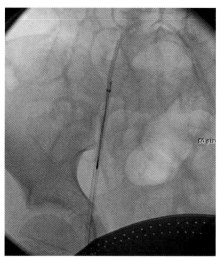

Figure 4.6

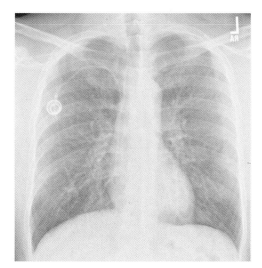

Findings

▶ A double-lumen, left-sided implantable venous access device (IVAD) is seen over the chest wall, but the catheter (arrowheads) is discontigous from the reservoir (arrow).

▶ A sheath is seen in the right atrium placed from a right common femoral vein approach (Fig. 4.4).
A gooseneck snare (arrow) has been tightened around the fractured catheter fragment, which was then removed through the sheath (Fig. 4.5).

▶ In a different patient (Fig. 4.6), a right-sided subclavian IVAD is seen, with narrowing of the catheter at the thoracic outlet representing impending fracture.

Teaching Points

▶ "Pinch-off syndrome" is a complication specific to subclavian vein access. Repetitive trauma from motion within costoclavicular space results in catheter fatigue and ultimately fracture. The costoclavicular space is bounded anteriorly by the clavicle, subclavius muscle, and costocoroacoid ligament; posteriorly by the first rib and the anterior scalene muscle; and medially by the costoclavicular ligament. This complication can be avoided by using the internal jugular vein approach.

▶ Pain with injection of a port is usually associated with either malpositon of the access (Huber) needle or extravasation from a hole in or discontinuity of the catheter.

Management

▶ When pain on injection of an IVAD occurs, the management algorithm should include (1) reaccess to exclude a malpositioned access needle; (2) evaluation of recent chest imaging to confirm position and continuity of the catheter; and (3) contrast study of the port to evaluate for leak.

▶ When identified, discontiguous catheter fragments should be removed as soon as possible to avoid secondary complications of free fragments in the heart or pulmonary arteries, including arrythmia and thrombosis.

▶ Removal may be performed from either a jugular or common femoral vein approach. In some cases, a tip-deflecting wire may be helpful to optimize positioning of the fragment for removal.

Further Reading

Mirza B, Vanek VW, Kupensky DT. Pinch-off syndrome: case report and collective review of the literature. *Am Surg.* 2004; *70*(7):635–644.

History

▶ A 56-Year-Old Man with End-Stage Renal Disease Presents with Preoperative Imaging Prior to Fistula Placement

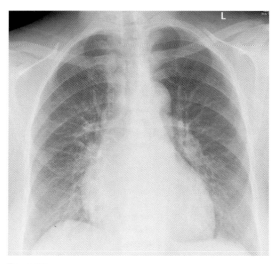

Figure 5.1

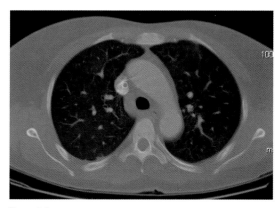

Figure 5.2

Case 5 Calcified Fibrin Sheath

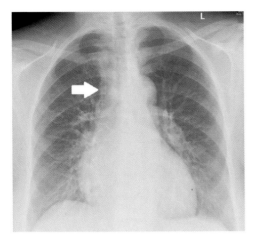

Figure 5.3

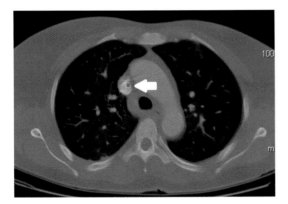

Figure 5.4

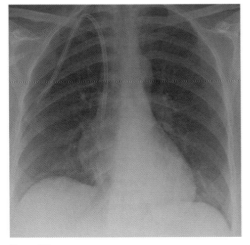

Figure 5.5

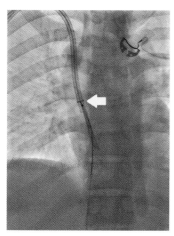

Figure 5.6

Findings

▶ A calcified tubular structure (white arrow) is seen (Fig. 5.3) overlying the superior vena cava.
▶ On computed tomography (CT) (Fig. 5.4) this tubular structure is shown to be within the superior vena cava (white arrow) representing a calcified fibrin sheath.
▶ A chest radiograph of the same patient prior to maturation of his dialysis fistula confirms the presence of a previous dialysis catheter (Fig. 5.5).

Teaching Points

▶ Fibrin sheaths are composed of fibrin and other coagulation factors that can cover a foreign body within hours of placement. If there is opposition to a vein wall, this film can further mature with addition of collagen and smooth muscle cells eventually leading to catheter malfunction.
▶ Catheters surrounded by fibrin sheaths can usually be injected, but blood cannot be aspirated.
▶ Over time, fibrin sheaths can calcify and can be misinterpreted as a foreign body.

Management

▶ Initial management of malfunctioning catheters involves injection of a low-dose fibrinolytic (alteplase) into each catheter lumen allowing a dwell time up to 90 minutes. While this can salvage up to 90% of catheters, patency is usually short term.
▶ Catheters positioned in the superior vena cava above the cavoatrial junction are at higher risk for fibrin sheath formation because close proximity to the vessel wall promotes deposition of muscle cells to the tip of the catheter.
▶ In dialysis patients, development of a fibrin sheath determines the long-term catheter patency. To maintain catheter patency, current guidelines of the American Society of Diagnostic and Interventional Nephrology Clinical Practice Committee recommend flushing (locking) after each use with either 1000 U/mL heparin or 4% trisodium citrate.
▶ More invasive techniques for catheter salvage include catheter stripping (Fig. 5.6; white arrow shows an endovascular snare around the hemodialysis catheter used to disrupt the sheath) or catheter exchange with or without balloon disruption of the fibrin sheath. If catheter exchange is chosen, a new venous puncture may be considered to avoid placing the new catheter into the same fibrin sheath.

Further Reading

Heye S, Maleux G, Goossens GA, et al. Feasibility and safety of endovascular stripping of totally implantable venous access devices. *Cardiovasc Interv Radiol*. 2012; 35:607–612.
Lu A, Smith DC. Calcified fibrin sheath masquerading as retained catheter. *J Vasc Interv Radiol*. 2013; 24:691.
Nayeemuddin M, Pherwani AD, Asquith JR. Imaging and management of complications of central venous catheters. *Clin Radiol*. 2013; 68:529–544.

History

▶ High Output from Chest Tube for 10 Days Following Esophagectomy for Early-Stage Carcinoma. What is the Diagnosis and What Procedure is Being Performed?

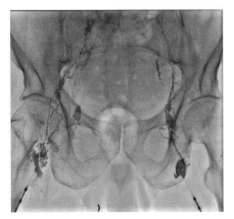

Figure 6.1

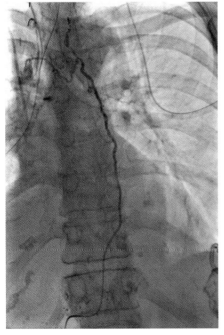

Figure 6.2

Case 6   Lymphangiogram and Thoracic Duct Embolization

Figure 6.3

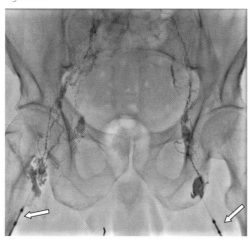

Figure 6.4

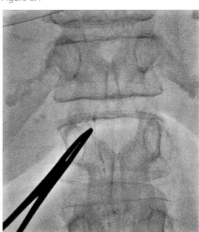

Figure 6.5

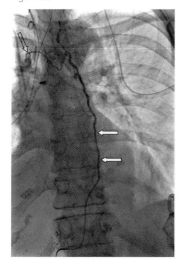

Figure 6.6

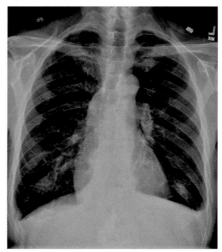

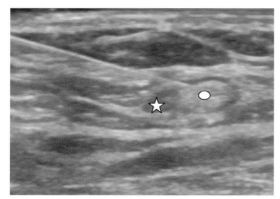

Figure 6.7

Findings

▶ Bilateral groin lymph nodes have been accessed with 25-gauge needles (Fig. 6.3, arrows). Ethiodol has been injected and is opacifying pelvic lymphatics.

▶ Contrast is seen in the cysterna chyli (Fig. 6.4) identified at the tip of the clamp.

▶ After direct puncture of the cysternal chyle, a microcatheter has been placed into the thoracic duct (arrows). Contrast injected into the microcatheter demonstrates extravasation at the T2 vertebral level (hollow arrow).

▶ Three days after embolization with a mixture of Ethiodol and n-cyanoacrylate, chest X-ray (Fig. 6.6) shows a persistent cast of the embolic agent in the thoracic duct.

Teaching Points

▶ Chylous pleural effusions may result from trauma (most commonly iatrogenic at surgery) or due to occlusion of the thoracic duct, resulting in formation of leaky collaterals.

▶ Thoracic duct embolization was described as an alternative to surgical ligation. In early experience abdominal lymphatics were opacified after catheterization of tiny lymphatic channels in the dorsum of the foot that were opacified by subcutaneous injection of 1% isosulfan blue. With this technique, opacification of the cysterna chyle took several hours to days.

▶ Unlike pedal lymphathic catheterization, intranodal injection for lymphangiogram, performed in the current case, does not require special equipment and the cysterna chyle can usually be seen within 2 hours. Intranodal lymphangiography is performed by advancing a needle into a normal lymph node at the interface of the cortex (Fig. 6.7 star) and fatty hilum (Fig. 6.7 dot) and slowly injecting ethiodol. A total of 5–10 cc is usually sufficient.

▶ The cysterna chyle is most often at the L1-L2 level anterior to the spine and to the right of the aorta. After opacification it can be punctured percutaneously from an anterior approach and catheterized with a microcatheter.

▶ Lymphangiogram alone may be successful in treating some patients with chylous effusion or ascites. Embolization of the cysterna chyle is not, however, useful in treating patients with chylous ascites alone.

Management

▶ After identification of the leak, embolization of the thoracic duct distal and proximal to the extravasation using a combination of coils and n-butyl cyanoacrylate/Ethiodol may be performed. Ethiodol both opacifies and slows polymerization of the glue. Because glue polymerizes when in contact with ionic solution, the catheter should be flushed with sterile water prior to injecting the mixture.

▶ If the thoracic duct cannot be catheterized, maceration of the cysterna chyle with a 20- to 22-gauge needle may be performed with moderate success.

Further Reading

Chen E, Itkin M. Thoracic duct embolization for chylous leaks. *Semin Intervent Radiol.* 2011; 28:63–74.

Nadolski GJ, Itkin M. Feasibility of ultrasound guided intranodal lymphangiogram for thoracic duct embolization. *J Vasc Interv Radiol.* 2012; 23:613–616.

History

▶ A 59-year-old female smoker presented to her pulmonologist with a cough. Routine chest radiograph identified a nodule within her right lower lobe, prompting a computed tomography (CT) scan. Follow-up CT after completing a course of antibiotics reveals persistence of this nodule. You are asked to biopsy it. In recovery, the patient complains of shortness of breath.

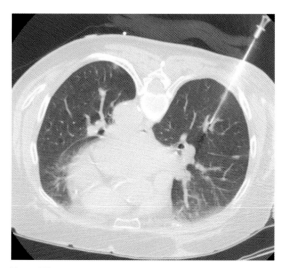

Figure 7.1

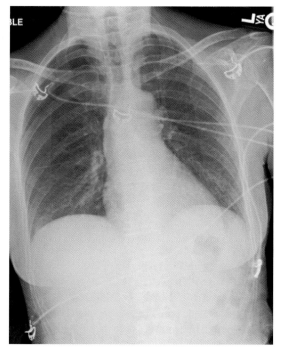

Figure 7.2

Case 7   Postbiopsy Pneumothorax

Figure 7.3

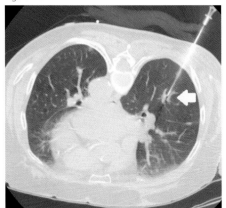

Figure 7.4

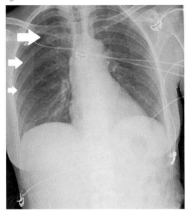

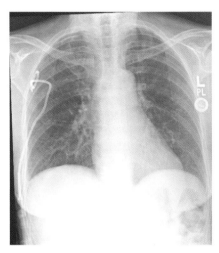

Figure 7.5

Findings

► A single image from the intraprocedural CT (Fig. 7.3) demonstrates a 20-gauge biopsy needle with the target lesion.
► On the chest radiograph obtained immediately after the biopsy (not shown) no pneumothorax was seen. A second radiograph (Fig. 7.4) obtained when the patient complained of acute shortness of breath in the recovery room demonstrates a moderate sized pneumothorax (arrows).
► After placement of a right thoracostomy tube (Fig. 7.5) there is re-expansion of the right lung.

Teaching Points

► While some of the risk factors associated with post biopsy pneumothoraces are controversial, universally accepted risks include degree of emphysema and number of pleural punctures (number of fissures crossed). Prior surgery, in the ipsilateral chest is considered protective. Recovering patients with the biopsy side in a dependent position and prone position during biopsy have also been suggested to be protective.
► Coaxial technique for biopsy is preferred by some because this technique minimizes the number of pleural punctures and affords the operator the ability to aspirate a pneumothorax should one be detected at the time of biopsy.

► Risk of pneumothorax after a lung biopsy ranges from 5% to 60%, with most recent literature suggesting a rate of 15%–25%. Approximately 5%–15% of patients will require a chest tube to treat post biopsy pneumothoraces.

Management

► While management of a pneumothorax varies by institution, we will recover and monitor patients for 2 hours after a routine lung biopsy. A chest radiograph is obtained within a few minutes after leaving the procedure room with a second chest radiograph obtained 2 hours after the procedure. A repeat radiograph should be obtained for symptoms of new or increased shortness of breath or increasing pleuritic pain (as in this case).

► Patients without a pneumothorax after the 2-hour recovery period are discharged home.

► A thoracostomy tube is placed for an enlarging pneumothorax or in symptomatic patients.

► There is tremendous variation in management of postlung biopsy chest tubes, ranging from an overnight hospital stay to outpatient management. When the lung remains expanded and there is no detectable air leak, the catheter may be clamped for a 2- to 4-hour trial. If at the end of this period there is no pneumothorax, the catheter may be safely removed.

► Pneumothoraces identified during the biopsy may be treated with manual aspiration alone, although aspiration of >500 cc is associated with a high likelihood of requiring chest tube placement.

Further Reading

Brown KT, Brody LA, Getrajdman GI, et al. Outpatient treatment of iatrogenic pneumothorax after needle biopsy. *Radiology*. 1997; *205*(1):249–252.

Cham MD, Lane ME, Henschke CI, et al. Lung biopsy: Special techniques. *Semin Respir Crit Care Med*. 2008; *29*:335–349.

MacMahon H, Austin JHM, Gamsu G, et al. Guidelines for management of small pulmonary nodules detected on CT scans: a statement from the Fleischner society. *Radiology*. 2005; *237*:395–400.

History

▶ A 74-Year-Old Male Status Post Resection of a Left Upper Lobe Non–Small Cell Lung Cancer with New Anteroposterior Window Lymph Node on Computed Tomography Requiring Biopsy

Is there a window to this lesion that avoids lung parenchyma?

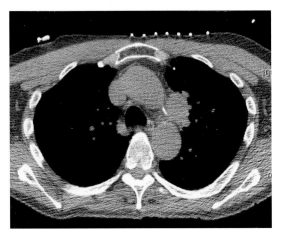

Figure 8.1

Case 8   Mediastinal Biopsy Utilizing Separation Techniques

Figure 8.2

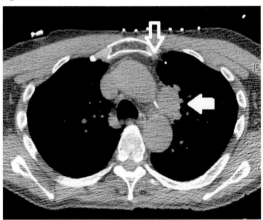

Figure 8.3

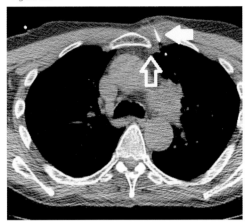

Figure 8.4

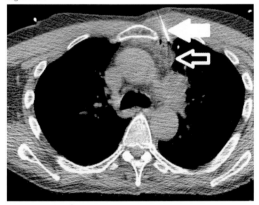

Figure 8.5

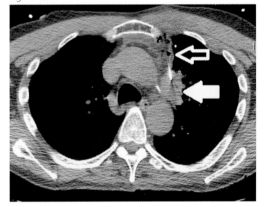

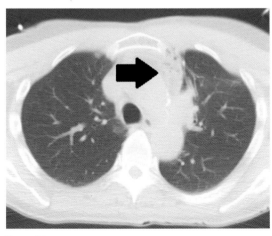

Figure 8.6

Findings

▶ Figure 8.2 demonstrates the target lymph node in station 5/6, also known as the AP window/paraaortic nodal station (white solid arrow).

▶ Figure 8.3 demonstrates a needle advanced into the mediastinal soft tissues (white solid arrow), just lateral to the mammary vessels (hollow white arrow in Figs. 8.2 and 8.3).

▶ Computed tomography (CT) after injection of 30 cc of normal saline was infused (Fig. 8.4) into the mediastinal space (hollow white arrow), creating an artificial window to advance the biopsy needle (solid white arrow) without traversing lung.

▶ After additional saline was infused to expand the potential space between the visceral and parietal pleura (hollow white arrow,) the biopsy needle was advanced into the target lymph node (Fig. 8.5, solid white arrow).

▶ Following the biopsy, lung window CT shows no pneumothorax (Fig. 8.6). Residual saline in the mediastinal soft tissues (black arrow) resolves within a few days.

Teaching Points

▶ Biopsy of mediastinal lymph nodes is typically done via endobronchial ultrasound or mediastinoscopy. Certain lymph node stations, however, are hard to target by these means. Station 5/6 is particularly difficult to access secondary to its proximity to the aorta and pulmonary artery.

▶ Percutaneous access of this location is typically done through lung parenchyma, and it is therefore associated with the risk of pneumothorax. Saline infusion into the pleural space can create an artificial window, allowing the biopsy to be performed without puncture of the visceral pleura.

▶ Knowledge of anatomy in this area is paramount to ensure internal mammary arteries (Figs. 8.2 and 8.3, hollow white arrow) are not inadvertently crossed.

Management

▶ Patients should be counseled as though a lung biopsy was performed; that is, watch for dyspnea, chest pain, or shoulder pain.

▶ Saline will resorb spontaneously, and it does not need to be aspirated at the end of the procedure.

Further Reading

Walker CM, Chung JH, Abbott GF, et al. Mediastinal lymph node staging: from noninvasive to surgical. *Am J Roentengenol.* 2012; 199:W54–W64.

History

▶ A 41-year-old male with a history of nephrolithiasis presents to the emergency department with abdominal pain. A computed tomography (CT) scan partially demonstrates a large mediastinal mass. Evaluate for potential of biopsy for diagnosis.

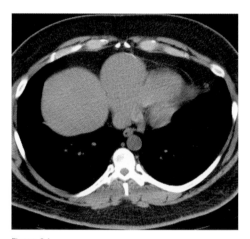

Figure 9.1

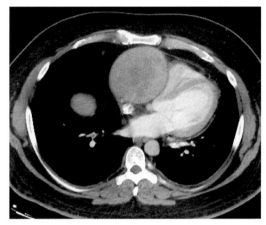

Figure 9.2

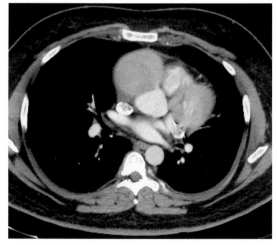

Figure 9.3

Case 9   Right Coronary Artery Aneurysm

Figure 9.4

Figure 9.5

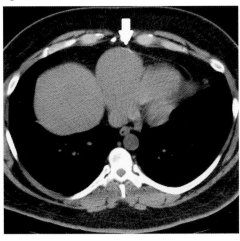
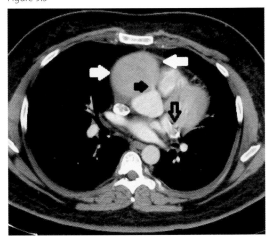

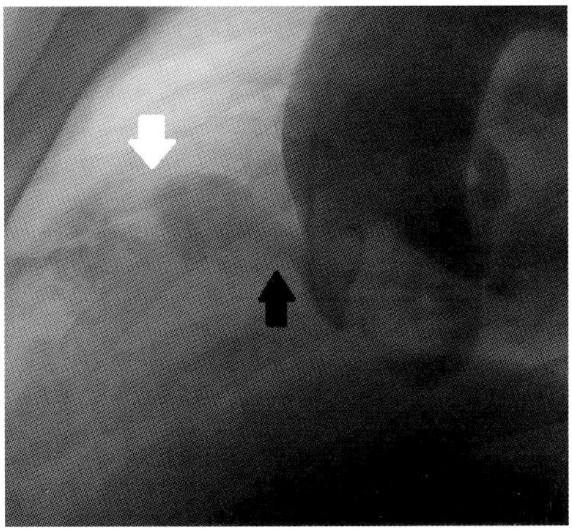

Figure 9.6

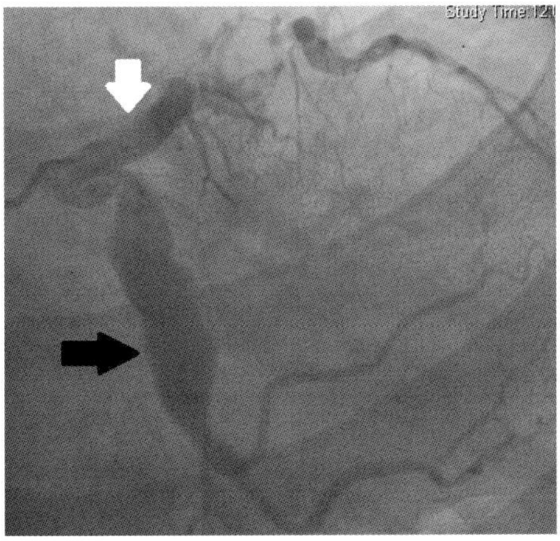

Figure 9.7

Findings

▸ A large mediastinal mass is identified on a noncontrast CT scan, which enhances with contrast administration (Figs. 9.4 and 9.5, white arrows). Peripheral calcification is identified along the walls of this mass anteriorly (Fig. 9.4, white arrow).

▸ Careful inspection of the postcontrast CT (Fig. 9.5) demonstrates a calcified aneurysm of the left circumflex coronary artery (open arrow) as well as contrast communicating between the aorta and mediastinal mass (black arrow), making the diagnosis of coronary artery aneurysm likely.

▸ Aortogram with the pigtail catheter in the aortic root (Fig. 9.6) shows contrast swirling (black arrow) in a large right coronary artery aneurysm (white arrow).

▸ Selective left main arteriogram (Fig. 9.7) demonstrates left circumflex (black arrow) and anterior descending artery (white arrow) aneurysms.

Teaching Points

▸ While this mass is easily accessible to biopsy, it is important to keep a vascular etiology in mind when evaluating a patient for potential biopsy. Here, clues include peripheral calcification and aneurysms of the other coronary arteries.

▶ Potential etiologies of coronary artery aneursyms include atherosclerosis, iatrogenic origin, infection, connective tissue disorders (Marfan's syndrome), vasculitis, or congenital causes such as Kawasaki's disease.

Management

▶ Complications of untreated aneuryms include rupture or distal embolization, causing ischemia and infarction.

▶ Asymptomatic patients are generally treated with anticoagulation and antiplatelet therapy.

▶ Symptomatic patients or those with large aneurysms (such as this case) are treated with coronary artery bypass with aneurysm exclusion or stent placement.

▶ The patient presented was treated with resection of the right coronary artery aneurym and a three-vessel coronary artery bypass.

Further Reading

Ebina T, Ishikawa Y, Uchida K, et al. A case of giant coronary artery aneurysm and literature review. *J Cardiol*. 2009; *53*:293–300.

Nichols L, Lagana S, Parwani A. Coronary artery aneurysm: A review and hypothesis regarding etiology. *Arch Pathol*. 2008; *132*:823–828.

History

▶ Positron Emission Tomography Scan Performed in the Workup of Newly Diagnosed Breast Cancer

Biopsy of this solitary positron emission tomography (PET) positive lesion was requested.

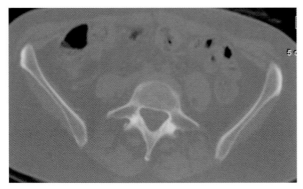

Figure 10.1

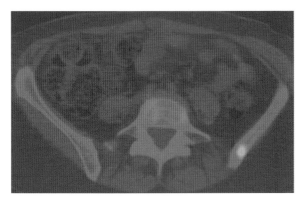

Figure 10.2

Case 10 Positron Emission Tomography–Guided Biopsy

Figure 10.3

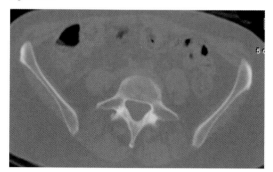

Figure 10.4

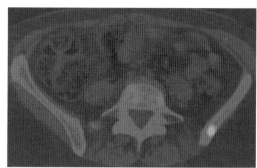

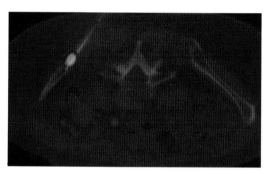

Figure 10.5

Findings

▶ A focus of fluorodeoxyglucose (FDG) activity is seen in the posterior left iliac bone (Fig. 10.4) that does not have a correlate on the computed tomography (CT) from the same level (Fig. 10.3).

▶ Using positron emission tomography (PET) guidance, a core biopsy needle is show within the PET avid left iliac bone lesion (Fig. 10.5). Pathology confirmed the presence of a metastasis from the patient's known breast cancer.

Teaching Points

▶ PET imaging is useful to target lesions that are FDG avid, but without imaging correlate on other cross-sectional imaging modalities more typically used for biopsy. Another use for PET-guided biopsy is to target the FDG avid regions of a lesion with heterogeneous activity.

▶ In this case, previous biopsy performed using landmarks was nondiagnostic. Bone marrow lesions are usually quite visible on magnetic resonance (MR), and this lesion could have more easily been sampled under MR guidance. However, this patient had a brain aneurysm coil precluding MR.

▶ When molecular diagnostics (e.g., EGFR, KRAS, BRAF) are required, biopsy of soft tissue rather than bone is preferred because the process of decalcification is usually performed with strong inorganic acids that results in significant degradation of both DNA and RNA in the sample.

▶ Misregistration of the PET and CT images is common in the upper abdomen due to respiratory motion. In some cases, long breath holds facilitated by intubation to maximize coregistration may be used. This is not usually an issue for lesions in the pelvis.

Management

▶ For PET-guided biopsy, the radiotracer should be administered intravenously at least 45 minutes prior to obtaining images. Acquisition time varies widely; if breath hold is required, images can be obtained in under 2 minutes.

▶ The dose required for biopsy guidance is less than that of a diagnostic PET. At our institution we use a dose of 4–6 mCi, and acquisition time ranges from <2 minutes when breath hold is required to 20 minutes for more diagnostic quality images.

▶ The radiation emitted from the patient is extremely low, and pregnant staff do not need to take any specific precaution except to avoid contact with the patient's urine.

Further Reading

Ryan ER, Sofocleous CT, Schöder H, et al. Split-dose technique for FDG PET/CT-guided percutaneous ablation: a method to facilitate lesion targeting and to provide immediate assessment of treatment effectiveness. *Radiology*. 2013; *268*(1):288–295.

Venkatesan AM, Kadoury S, Abi-Jaoudeh N, et al. Real-time FDG PET guidance during biopsies and radiofrequency ablation using multimodality fusion with electromagnetic navigation. *Radiology*. 2011; *260*(3):848–856.

History

▶ Two Different Patients with Lung Cancer Status post Contralateral Lung Resection Presented for Biopsy of Adrenal Masses

How would you minimize the risk of pneumothorax in the remaining solitary lung?

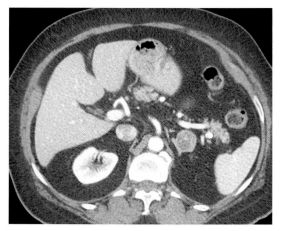

Figure 11.1

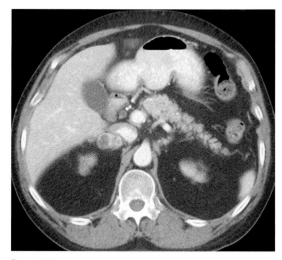

Figure 11.2

Case 11   Adrenal Biopsy

Figure 11.3

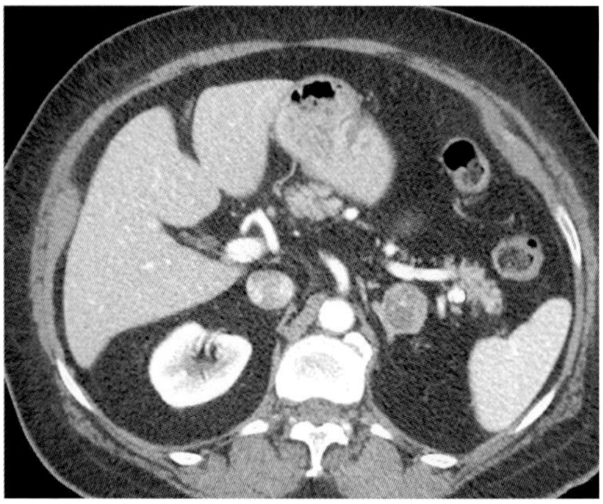

Figure 11.4

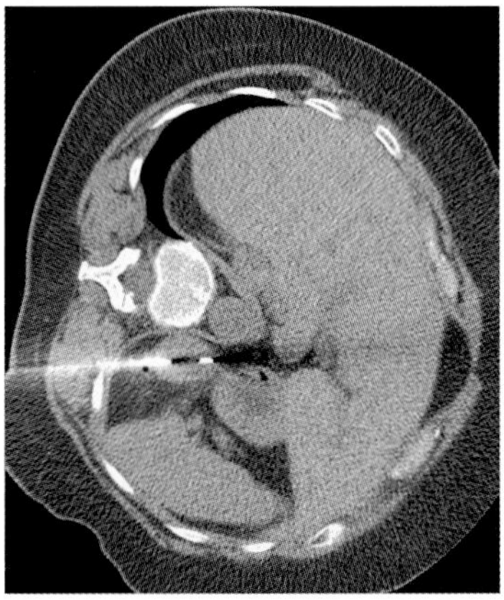

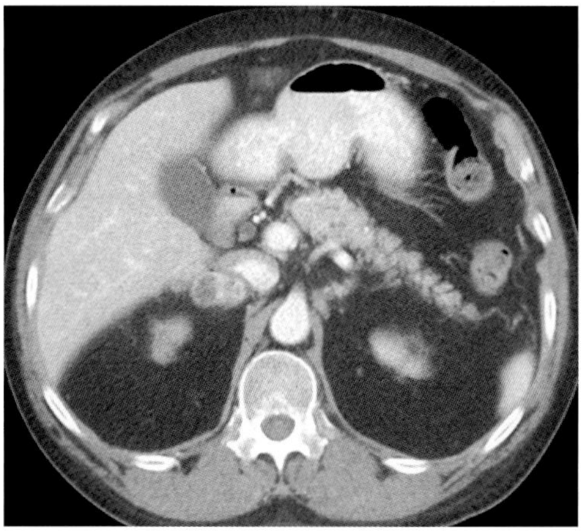

Figure 11.5

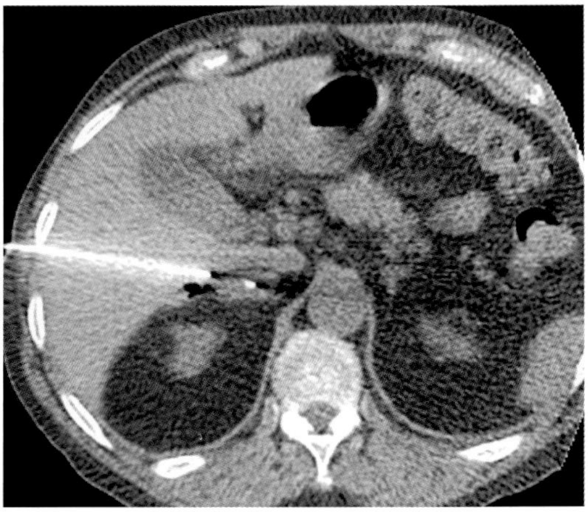

Figure 11.6

Findings

▶ Contrast-enhanced computed tomography (CT) images in two different patients demonstrate hypervascular lesions (Figs. 11.3 and 11.5) with areas of central necrosis in the left and right adrenal gland, respectively.

▶ In the first patient, left-side-down decubitous position (Fig. 11.4) was used to perform core biopsy. In this position, the needle has been advanced into the left adrenal gland avoiding aerated lung. Note that the nondependent right lung is seen at the same level.

▶ A transhepatic approach to adrenal biopsy was successfully performed in the patient with the right adrenal mass (Fig. 11.6).

Teaching Points

▶ If adrenal adenoma, which occurs in 2%–8% based on autopsy studies, is considered in the differential of an adrenal lesion, dedicated adrenal imaging with multiphase CT or magnetic resonance (MR) may clinch the diagnosis without the need for biopsy.

▶ Prior to biopsy of adrenal mass, consideration should be given to the possiblity of a catecholamine-producing pheochromocytoma. Pheochromocytoma follow the "rule of 10": 10% malignant, 10% bilateral, 10% extraadrenal, and 10% hereditary.

- There are several approaches to adrenal biopsy. Prone position is very common but has an increased risk of transpleural needle pass and resulting pneumothorax (even when there is no interposition of lung seen on the prebiopsy, supine CT). Ipsilateral-side-down decubitus compresses the lung and in some cases can be used to avoid pleural puncture and the risk of pneumothorax. To access right adrenal lesions, a transhepatic approach may be considered. Alternatively, a subdiaphragmatic approach may be performed with the patient prone using ultrasound or MR, or by tilting the CT gantry.

Management

- If pheochromocytoma is in the differential, 24-hour urine catecholamines should be performed prior to biopsy. If elevated and a biopsy is still indicated, pretreatment with alpha blockade should be considered to avoid hypertensive crisis.
- Because the adrenal gland is a common site of metastatic disease, biopsy of the adrenal tumor (as opposed to the suspected primary) has the potential to provide information for staging as well as tissue diagnosis. There are some data to support that the diagnostic yield from biopsy of metastatic disease may be higher than that of the primary in lung cancer.

Further Reading

Tam AL, Kim ES, Lee JJ, et al. Feasibility of image-guided transthoracic core-needle biopsy in the BATTLE lung trial. *J Thorac Oncol*. 2013; *8*(4):436–442.

Thompson GB, Young WF Jr. Adrenal incidentaloma. *Curr Opin Oncol*. 2003; *15*(1):84–90.

History

▶ A 62-Year-Old Female with Postprandial Pain

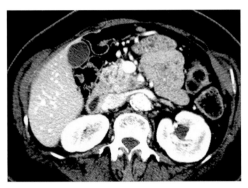

Figure 12.1

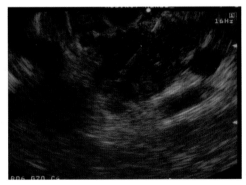

Figure 12.2

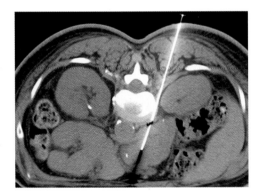

Figure 12.3

Case 12 Transcaval Pancreatic Biopsy

Figure 12.4

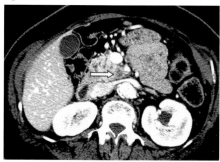

Figure 12.5

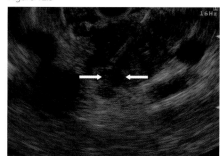

Figure 12.6

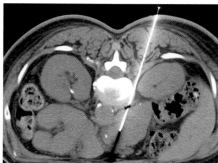

Figure 12.7

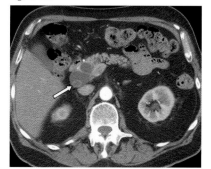

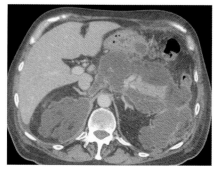

Figure 12.8

Findings

- A single image from a contrast-enhanced computed tomography (CT) (Fig. 12.4) shows a 1.2 cm mass in the uncinate process of the pancreas (arrow).
- Endoscopic ultrasound-guided biopsy of the mass (arrows) was performed (Fig. 12.5) but yielded a nondiagnostic specimen.
- Percutaneous needle biopsy using a posterior transcaval approach (Fig. 12.6) clinched the diagnosis of pancreatic cancer.
- CT from a different patient with a cystic pancreatic head mass (Fig. 12.7) with an enhancing mural nodule (arrow) who subsequently underwent endoscopic ultrasound-guided biopsy. Several days following biopsy the patient complained of abdominal pain, and a second CT was performed (Fig. 12.8) demonstrating acute pancreatitis with multiple developing pseudocysts. Biopsy confirmed a branch duct intraductal pancreatic mucinous neoplasm.

Teaching Points

▶ Pancreatic biopsy may be performed using endoscopic ultrasound guidance. Compared to percutaneous biopsy, endoscopic biopsy has higher yield for small lesions, may detect peripancreatic lymph nodes, and minimizes the risk of tract seeding (see Case 103). However, this technique is highly operator dependent and not all lesions are accessible.

▶ Fine-needle aspiration biopsy of uncinate and pancreatic head masses may be safely performed using a transcaval approach. Alternatively, in some cases, an anterior transgastric approach may be possible.

▶ Complications include bleeding, tract seeding, and acute pancreatitis.

Management

▶ The need for preoperative biopsy in patients with resectable pancreatic masses is controversial. Indications for biopsy of a resectable lesion include diagnosing a lesion that would not be treated surgically, for example, lymphoma, focal autoimmune pancreatitis, or a pancreatic neuroendocrine tumor that potentially could be enucleated and not require a pancreaticoduodenectomy.

▶ Identification of the right renal artery should be made prior to biopsy to avoid inadvertent puncture of this vessel.

Further Reading

Sofocleous, CT, Schubert J, Brown KT, et al. CT-guided transvenous or transcaval needle biopsy of pancreatic and peripancreatic lesions. *J Vasc Interv Radiol.* 2004; *15*(10):1099–1104.

History

▶ Abdominal Pain and Jaundice Elevated Amylase and Lipase. What is the most likely diagnosis?

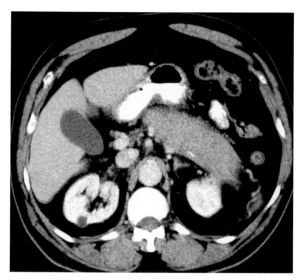

Figure 13.1

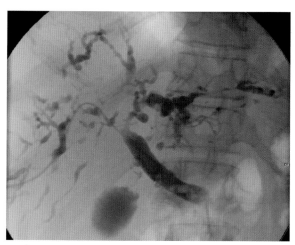

Figure 13.2

Case 13 Autoimmune Pancreatitis with Biliary Tract Involvement

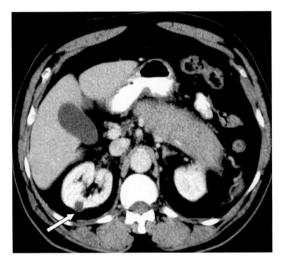

Figure 13.3

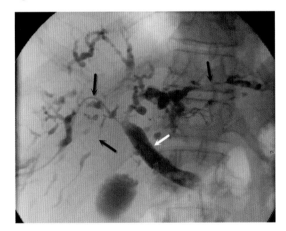

Figure 13.4

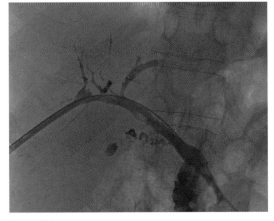

Figure 13.5

Findings

▶ Contrast-enhanced computed tomography (CT) (Fig. 13.3) shows an enlarged featureless pancreas without pancreatic duct dilation. There is a "halo" of low density at the periphery of the gland. Finally, a low-density lesion is seen in the right renal cortex (arrow).

▶ Percutaneous cholangiogram (Fig. 13.4) in a different patient with the same disease process shows multiple intrahepatic biliary strictures (black arrows) extending to the common duct (white arrow), which has a more normal appearance.

▶ After a course of oral steroid therapy (Fig. 13.5), the stenoses at the confluence are improved and the drainage catheter is removed.

Teaching Points

▶ Imaging findings of an edematous, featureless pancreas without ductal dilation should raise the possibilty of autoimmune pancreatitis. A "halo" of inflammatory changes is commonly seen at the periphery of the gland.

▶ Focal autoimmune pancreatitis can mimic pancreatic cancer. Typical symptoms include obstructive jaundice, abdominal pain, and type II diabetes.

▶ Extrahepatic manifestations of autoimmune pancreatitis (AIP) include biliary involvement and renal deposits, as in this case. Renal disease represents foci of cortical lymphoplasmocytic infiltrates. Retroperitoneal disease, salivary glands, and enlarged lymph nodes, as well as lesions in the lung and gastrointestinal tract, may also be present.

Management

▶ AIP is usually, but not always, associated with elevated serum IgG4. This, in combination with response to immune suppression, clinches the diagnosis.

▶ AIP is most commonly diffuse but may be focal. When AIP is considered in the differential of a pancreatic mass, immunohistochemistry stains for IgG4 can help differentiate a lesion from a neoplasm.

▶ The imaging appearance and function of the pancreas usually normalize 4–6 weeks into treatment.

Further Reading

Vlachou PA, Khalili K, Jang HJ, et al. IgG4 related sclerosing disease: Autoimmune pancreatitis and extrapancreatic manifestations. *Radiographics*. 2011; *31*:1379–1402.

History

▶ Post Bone Marrow Transplant, Thrombocytopenia with Elevated Liver Function Tests

Pressure measured with the catheter in Fig. 14.1 was 10 mmHg and in Fig. 14.2 was 24 mmHg. Right atrial pressure was 6–8 mmHg.

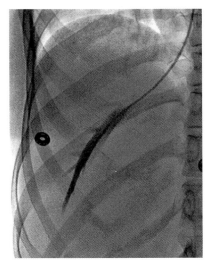

Figure 14.1

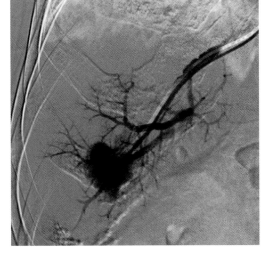

Figure 14.2

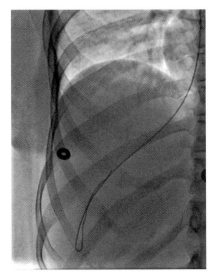

Figure 14.3

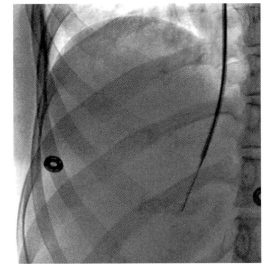

Figure 14.4

Case 14 Transjugular Liver Biopsy

Figure 14.5

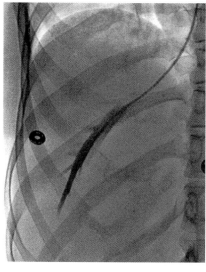

Figure 14.6

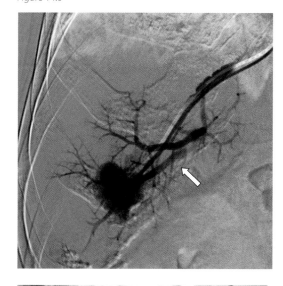

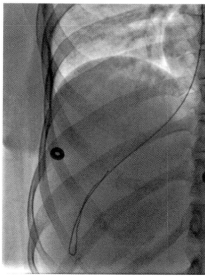

Figure 14.7

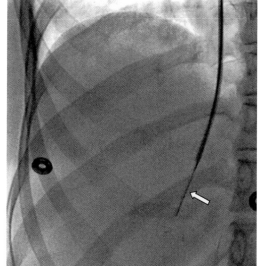

Figure 14.8

Findings

▶ Transjugular access of the right hepatic vein has been achieved via the right internal jugular vein approach (Fig. 14.5).

▶ In Figure 14.5 the end-hole catheter is positioned freely in the hepatic vein; in Figure 14.6 it is wedged in a terminal branch of the hepatic vein and contrast injected in this position opacifies the right portal vein branches (arrow).

▶ An 18-gauge side-notch biopsy needle has been advanced through the metallic sheath (arrow, Fig. 14.8) to obtain a random core of liver tissue.

Teaching Points

▶ Transjugular (vs. percutaneous) liver biopsy is indicated when a nontarget sample is required in patients with ascites or coagulopathy. It may also be performed in conjunction with other procedures requiring venous access, including hepatic venography or pressure measurements.

▶ The hepatic venous pressure gradient (HVPG) is calculated by subtracting the free hepatic vein pressure from the wedge pressure measurement which provides an indirect measurement of portal vein pressure. A normal value is less than 5 mmHg. In cirrhotic patients, varices typically develop at an HVPG over 10 mmHg.

▶ In Figure 14.7 an Amplatz wire has been advanced deep into the right hepatic vein so that the floppy tip is coiled distally. This provides a stiff wire along the entire course of access to facilitate placement of the metal cannula of the biopsy set.

▶ Because the central hepatic veins are posterior relative to the bulk of liver parenchyma, the metal sheath is rotated anteriorly to direct the biopsy needle into the parenchyma and to minimize the risk of capsular perforation.

▶ Multiple cores should be obtained and sent for appropriate studies. In the evaluation of cirrhosis, evaluation of fewer than three cores may underestimate stage. In select cases, specimens may be obtained for culture and/or quantitative iron analysis.

Management

▶ Repeated measurement of hepatic venous pressure gradient may be used to evaluate for response of portal pressure to beta blockade in patients with cirrhosis.

Further Reading

McAfee JH, Keeffe EB, Lee RG, et al. Transjugular liver biopsy. *J Hepatol.* 1992; 15(4):726–732.

Transjugular liver biopsy. In: Mauro MA, Murphy KPJ, Thomson KR, Venbrux AC, Zollikofer CL, eds. *Image-Guided Interventions*. Philadelphia, PA: Saunders; 2008:762–767.

History

▶ A 76-Year-Old Male with Hematuria and Pain 3 Days after Nontarget Kidney Biopsy

What is the most likely diagnosis and the appropriate management?

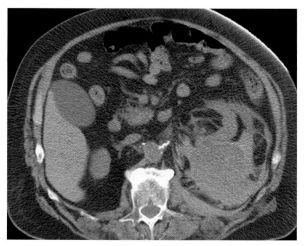

Figure 15.1

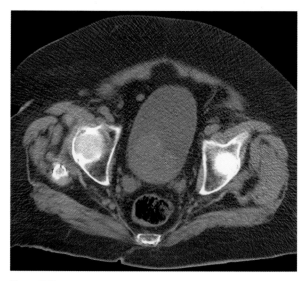

Figure 15.2

Case 15   Renal Pseudoaneurysm

Figure 15.3

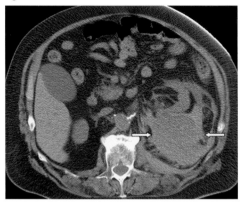

Figure 15.4

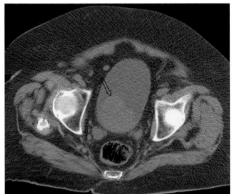

Figure 15.5

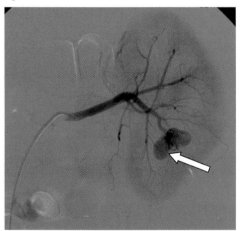

Figure 15.6

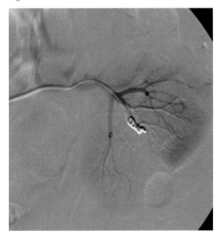

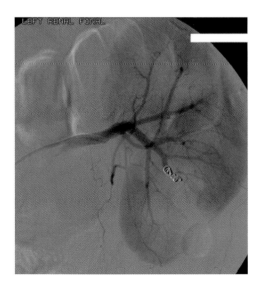

Figure 15.7

Findings

▶ Noncontrast computed tomography (CT) 3 days after biopsy (Figs. 15.3 and 15.4) demonstrates a large left perinephric hematoma (arrows) and dense clot within the bladder (hollow arrow).

▶ Left renal angiogram (Fig. 15.5) demonstrates a pseudoaneurysm (arrow) arising from the lower pole renal artery in the area that was biopsied (not shown).

▶ After subselective coil embolization (Fig. 15.6), the pseudoaneurysm is no longer opacified and the majority of the renal arteries are preserved (Fig. 15.7).

Teaching Points

▶ Pseudoaneurysms of the renal arteries are commonly the sequela of trauma, most often iatrogenic following renal biopsy, nephrostomy placement, or partial nephrectomy.

▶ The constellation of persistent hematuria and bleeding around the catheter following nephrostomy should raise the possibility of pseudoaneurysm.

Management

▶ Most iatrogenic pseudoaneuryms involve distal subsegmental branches of the renal artery. The classic teaching for embolization of pseudoaneurysms is to embolize with permanent agent (e.g., coils) both proximal and distal to the injury to prevent collateral reperfusion. In these very distal arteries this is not usually possible, and proximal embolization suffices.

▶ Unlike in a true aneurysm, in which packing the aneurysm to preserve the native vessel is effective treatment, packing of a pseudoaneurysm, for example with coils, should be avoided because pseudoaneurysms represent contained ruptures and packing can increase pressure and promote free rupture.

▶ Permanent embolic agents, including thrombin, coils, glue, and particles, have been used to treat these lesions. Occasionally pseudoaneurysms are seen in association with renal arterio-venous fistula. In such cases particles should not be used because of the risk of shunting to the pulmonary arteries.

▶ Patients may experience a postembolization syndrome consisting of pain, nausea, and fever. Adverse effect on renal function or hypertension is uncommon.

Further Reading

Sildiroglu O, Saad WE, Hagspiel KD, et al. Endovascular management of iatrogenic native renal arterial pseudoaneurysms. *Cardiovasc Intervent Radiol.* 2012; 35(6):1340–1345.

History

▶ Retroperitoneal sarcoma was resected 2 years ago. New perineal mass is suspicious for recurrence. Biopsy was requested.

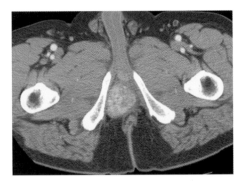

Figure 16.1

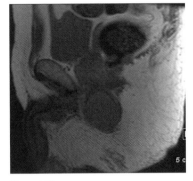

Figure 16.2

Case 16 Transperineal Magnetic Resonance–Guided Biopsy

Figure 16.3

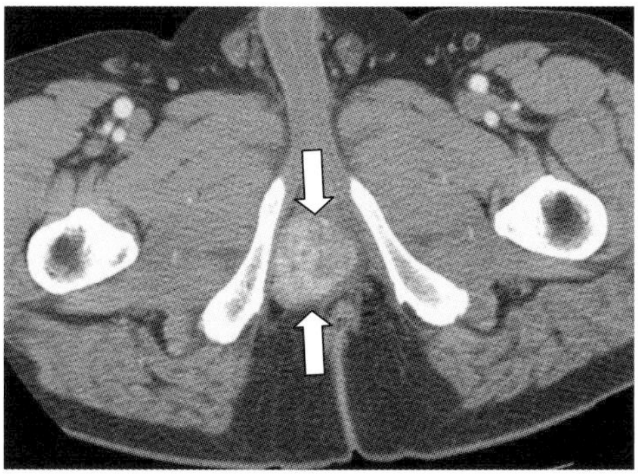

Figure 16.4

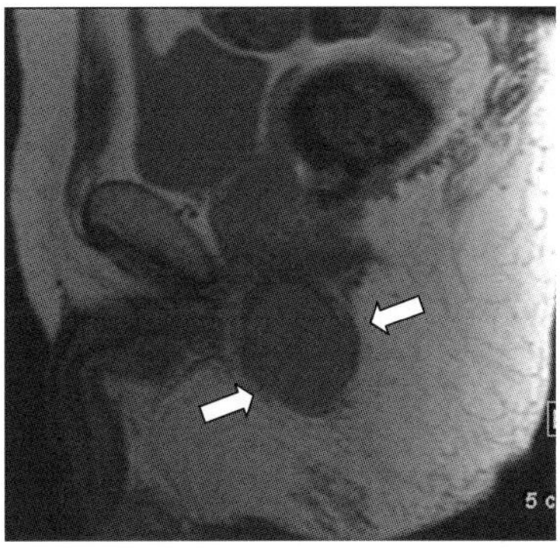

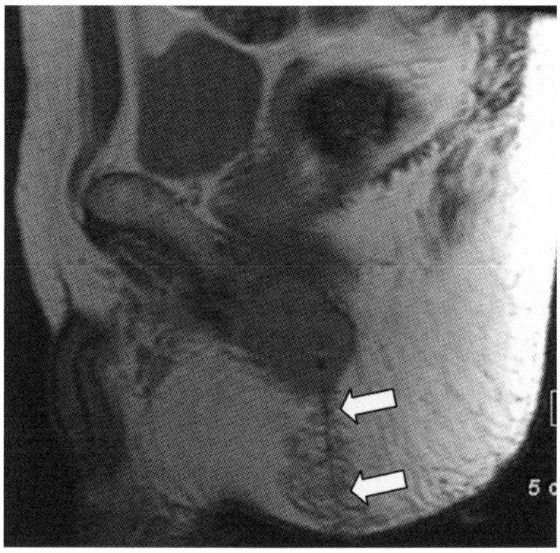

Figure 16.5

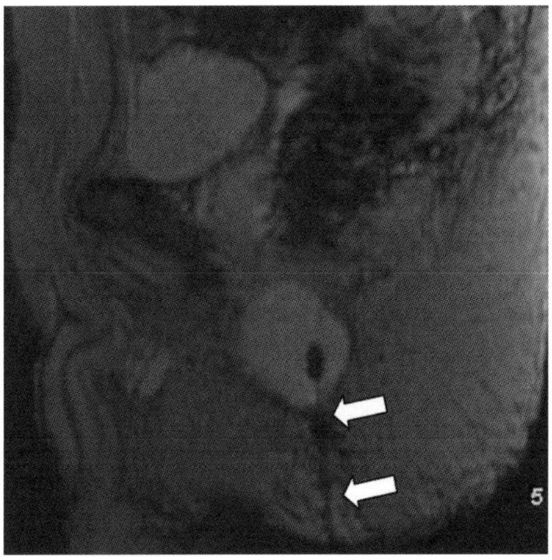

Figure 16.6

Findings

▶ Contrast-enhanced computed tomography (CT) shows an enhancing mass in the ishiorectal fossa (Fig. 16.3). Prebiopsy sagittal T2-weighted proton density magnetic resonance (MR) also shows the mass (Fig. 16.4).

▶ T1- and T2-weighted sagittal MR images (Figs. 16.5 and 16.6) show an MR-compatible biopsy needle within the mass from a transperineal approach.

Teaching Points

▶ Advantages of MR guidance for select biopsies include its superior soft tissue contrast (e.g., bone marrow lesions) and multiplanar capabilities allowing a biopsy trajectory in almost any plane.

▶ Several factors contribute to needle visualization, including sequence, field strength, needle composition, and direction of the frequency encoding direction. In general, artifact is increased with faster sequences, higher field strength, and imaging perpendicular to the frequency encoding direction. Blooming artifact at the needle tip (Fig. 16.4, arrowhead) occurs when the needle is parallel to the static magnetic field.

▶ Biopsy approach to potentially resectable bone and soft tissue tumors (sarcoma) should be discussed with the surgeon. Because of the high incidence of tract seeding from these tumors, resection is planned so as to include the needle tract with the tumor en bloc. Transperineal biopsy in this case was based on the anticipated transperineal resection.

Management

► Because MR-compatable biopsy devices are made from nonferrous metals, including nickel, titanium, and chromium, they are more pliable and less sharp than their traditional ferromagnetic stainless steel counterparts.

► MR affords the ability to image in multiple planes using a variety of sequences to maximize lesion and needle conspicuity.

Further Reading

Schwartz HS, Spengler DM. Needle tract recurrences after closed biopsy for sarcoma: three cases and review of the literature. *Ann Surg Oncol.* 1997; *4*(3):228–236.

Weiss CR, Nour SG, Lewin JS. MR guided biopsy: A review of current techniques and applications. *J Magn Reson Imaging.* 2008; *27*:311–325.

History

► Pancreatic Cancer with Intractable Back Pain

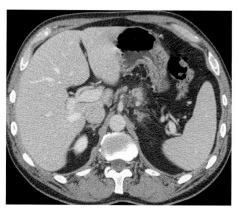

Figure 17.1

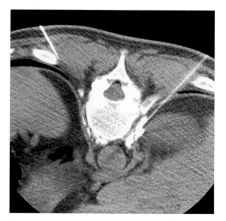

Figure 17.2

Case 17 Celiac Plexus Neurolysis

Figure 17.3

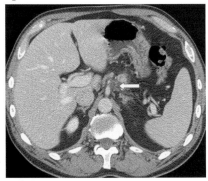

Figure 17.4

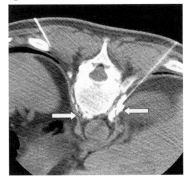

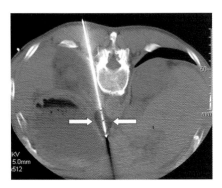

Figure 17.5

Findings

▶ Contrast-enhanced abdominal computed tomography (CT) image shows the level of the celiac plexus, which lays anterior to the aorta just below the origin of the celiac axis. Note the soft tissue attenuation around the proximal celiac axis (Fig. 17.3, arrow) representing tumor infiltration from a pancreatic cancer.

▶ With the patient in the prone position, bilateral 22-gauge needles have been advanced to the celiac plexus (Fig. 17.4). Contrast-opacified ethanol has been injected for neurolysis (arrows) and is seen posterior to the diaphragmatic crus.

▶ In a different patient, unilateral cryoablation was used to perform celiac neurolysis (Fig. 17.5). The iceball can be seen as a low-density oval structure forming around the distal end of the cryoprobe (arrows).

Teaching Points

▶ "Neurolysis" refers to permanent destruction of nerve, whereas "nerve block" refers to temporary interruption of nerve signaling by steroids or anesthetics.

▶ Visceral pain related to pancreatic cancer arises via visceral afferent nerves that coalesce at the celiac plexus. Debilitating pain from intra-abdominal malignancies, most notably pancreatic cancer, can greatly limit quality of life. In many patients, neurolysis can provide relief.

▶ The celiac plexus receives stimuli from the distal esophagus to the transverse colon, including the pancreas. With high-quality imaging, the ganglia can be identified more often than not. The right ganglia may be discoid soft tissue attenuation between the inferior vena cava and crus of the diaphragm.

Management

▶ Celiac neurolysis may be achieved with endoscopic ultrasound guidance or percutaneously with CT guidance. CT has the advantage of being able to visualize the distribution of the injectate accurately—which should ideally be both antecrural and retrocrural.

▶ Most commonly used for malignancy, neurolysis has also been used to treat the pain associated with chronic pancreatitis.

▶ Ethanol is the most common agent used for neurolysis. On CT scan, ethanol is seen as fat density. Contrast mixed with an anesthetic may be injected prior to ethanol to confirm free diffusion of the injectate.

▶ Other approaches, including anterior and decubitus, have been described for patients who cannot maintain a prone position.

▶ Compliations include pain, orthostatic hypotension, and diarrhea due to splanchnic vasodilation.

Further Reading

Kambadakone A, Thabet A, Gervais DA, et al. CT-guided celiac plexus neurolysis: a review of anatomy, indications, technique and tips for successful treatment. *Radiographics*. 2011; *31*(6):1599–1621.

History

▶ A 47-Year-Old Female Presented with a History of Breast Cancer. Computed Tomography Was Performed for Abdominal Pain.

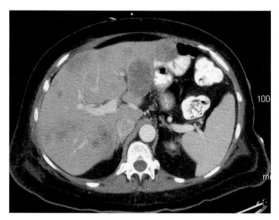

Figure 18.1

Case 18 Liver Biopsy

Figure 18.2

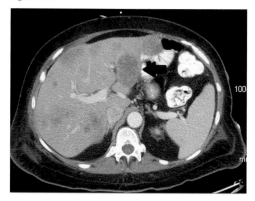

Figure 18.3

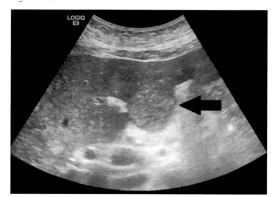

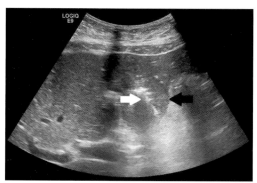

Figure 18.4

Findings

▶ Figure 18.2 demonstrates multiple hypodense lesions in the liver suspicious for metastasis. A lesion in segment 2/3 was targeted for biopsy (black arrow). It is important to choose a area to biopsy with the least amount of necrosis to increase yield.

▶ Ultrasound demonstrates the left hemiliver (Fig. 18.3, black arrow). When possible, choosing a path that traverses normal liver parenchyma may decrease the risk of bleeding.

▶ In Figure 18.4 the biopsy needle (white arrow) is seen within the target lesion (black arrow). When core biopsy is planned, it is important to take the throw of the biopsy needle (usually from 1 to 2cm) into account to avoid injury to structures deep to the biopsy target.

Teaching Points

▶ Image-guided liver biopsies are performed in a targeted fashion for focal lesions and in a nontargeted fashion to evaluate for parenchymal disease (see Case 14).

▶ For targeted liver lesions, the presence of on onsite cytopathology increases the diagnostic rate. If a cytopathologist is unavailable, three core biopsies allow for diagnosis in ~90% of cases.

▶ In a 2009 position paper, the American Association for the Study of Liver Diseases recommends a 16-gauge core biopsy be obtained to allow diagnosis, grading, and staging of diffuse, nonneoplastic parenchymal disease. In practice, many practitioners obtain 18- to 20-gauge core specimens.

Management

▶ Patients are observed in a recovery area for 2 to 4 hours. The majority of complications manifest within the first 2 hours.

▶ The most frequent major complication is bleeding that requires therapy—including transfusion, overnight observation, or embolization. Patients with major bleeding will manifest with pain refractory to pain medications with associated tachycardia, hypotension, and/or drop in hematocrit. There should be a low threshold to obtain urgent noncontrast computed tomography (CT) imaging of the abdomen if there is concern for bleeding.

Further Reading

Applebaum L, Kane RA, Kruskal JB, et al. Focal hepatic lesions: US guided biopsy—Lessons from review of cytologic and pathologic examination results. *Radiology*. 2009; *250*:453–458.

Vijayaraghavan GR, David S, Bermudez-Allende M, et al. Image-guided parenchymal liver biopsy: How we do it. *J Clin Imaging Sci*. 2011; *1*:1–8.

History

▶ A 25-Year-Old Female with Cold Intolerance. Workup for Hyperthyroidism Included an Ultrasound.

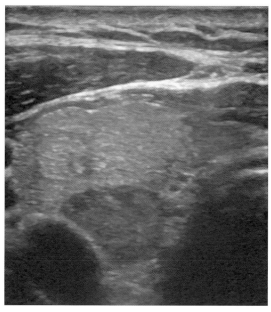

Figure 19.1

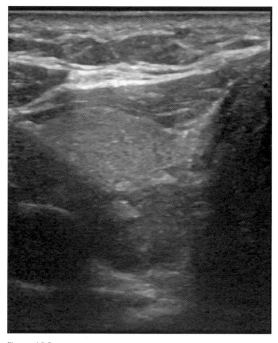

Figure 19.2

Case 19 Thyroid Biopsy

Figure 19.3

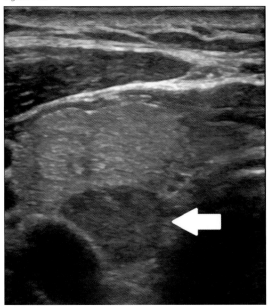

Figure 19.4

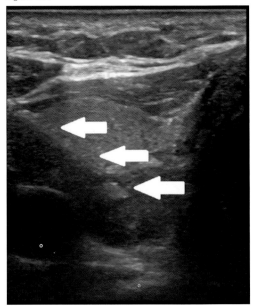

Findings

▶ A hypoechoic lesion (white arrow) is seen in the left thyroid lobe (Fig. 19.3) demonstrating vascularity (not shown).

▶ A 25-gauge biopsy needle (white arrows) is seen within the lesion (Fig. 19.4).

Teaching Points

▶ Different techniques have been used to obtain samples from thyroid biopsies, namely aspiration using suction or capillary action. Neither has proven to be superior and both are used clinically.

▶ Because of the small working area, it is easy to contaminate the specimen with ultrasound gel; to avoid this problem, either saline or betadine can be used as a coupling agent.

▶ When lesions are mixed cystic and solid, the solid component should be targeted for biopsy.

Management

▶ While the decision to biopsy certain thyroid nodules remains controversial, in 2009 the American Thyroid Association suggested certain guidelines in choosing which nodules to biopsy:

1. In patients without risk factors for thyroid cancer:
   ◾ All solid nodules greater than 1 cm in size with suspicious ultrasound characteristics.
      • Suspicious characteristics include the following:
         • Microcalcifications
         • Irregular borders or ill-defined margins
         • Cold on scintigraphy
   ◾ Mixed cystic and solid nodules without suspicious ultrasound features that are greater than 2.0 cm.
2. For patients with risk factors for thyroid cancer, nodule size threshold for biopsy decreases to 0.5 cm.

Further Reading

Frates MC, Benson CB, Charboneau JW, et al; Society of Radiologists in Ultrasound. Management of thyroid nodules detected at US: Society of radiologists in ultrasound consensus conference statement. *Radiology.* 2005; *237*:794–800.

Nixon IJ, Ganly I, Hann LE, et al. Nomogram for selecting thyroid nodules for ultrasound-guided fine-needle aspiration biopsy based on a quantification of risk of malignancy. *Head Neck.* 2013; *35*(7):1022–1025.

History

▶ A 69-Year-Old Female with Hepatocellular Carcinoma

Following multiple embolizations, residual and enlarging focus of viable disease is seen anteriorly in segment VIII. What is the procedure being performed?

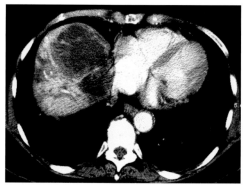

Figure 20.1

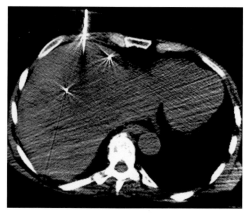

Figure 20.2

Case 20   Placement of Fiducial Markers to Facilitate Image-Guided Radiation Therapy

Figure 20.3

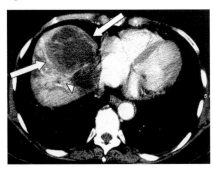

Figure 20.4

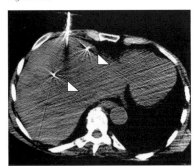

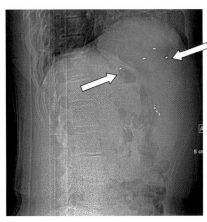

Figure 20.5

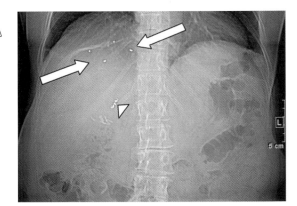

Figure 20.6

Findings

► A single image from a contrast-enhanced computed tomography (CT) scan shows a 6 cm viable tumor at the dome of the liver (Fig. 20.3, arrows). Posteriorly (arrowhead) is an area of treated tumor that had been stable for 18 months.

► Noncontrast CT at the time of fiducial marker placement (Fig. 20.4) shows two gold fiducial markers (arrowheads), one at the anterior medial border of the tumor and a second at the lateral aspect of the tumor. A needle is seen targeting a third location within the tumor for placement of an additional fiducial markers.

► Anteroposterior and lateral scout images from the treatment-planning CT (Figs. 20.5 and 20.6) show placement of four fiducial markers (arrows) in multiple superior/inferior and anterior/posterior positions relative to the tumor. Coils are present lower in the liver (arrowhead) from prior embolization of an arterio-portal shunt seen during a therapeutic embolization.

Teaching Points

▶ Image-guided radiation therapy (IGRT) is performed using orthogonal imaging to visualize opaque fiducial markers to provide precise targeting of the tumor during the entire treatment. This is most commonly indicated in areas susceptible to respiratory motion, including the lung and upper abdominal viscera.

▶ Fiducial markers placed within necrotic parts of tumors are prone to migrating within the tumor. This has also been an issue with fiducial markers placed in small lung lesions.

▶ Optimal placement involves placement of at least three markers in different planes within the tumor as seen on orthogonal imaging.

Management

▶ Fiducial markers can be made from gold or platinum. They are typically submillimeter in diameter and can be placed coaxially through an 18- or 19-gauge needle.

▶ As an alternative in lung, coils may be placed to minimize the risk of migration of markers out of the parenchyma and into the pleural space.

▶ When indicated, core biopsy can be performed through the access needle prior to fiducial implantation.

Further Reading

Kothary N, Dieterich S, Louie JD, et al. Percutaneous implantation of fiducial markers for imaging-guided radiation therapy. *Am J Roentgenol.* 2009; *192*:1090–1096.

History

▸ Hepatocellular Carcinoma in a Patient with Nonalcoholic Steatohepatitis

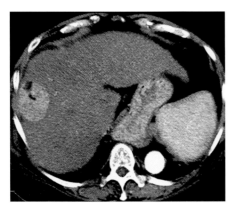

Figure 21.1

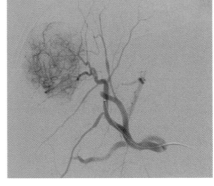

Figure 21.2

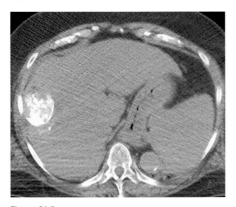

Figure 21.3

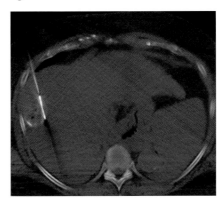

Figure 21.4

Case 21   Hepatocellular Carcinoma Treated with Microwave Ablation

Figure 21.5

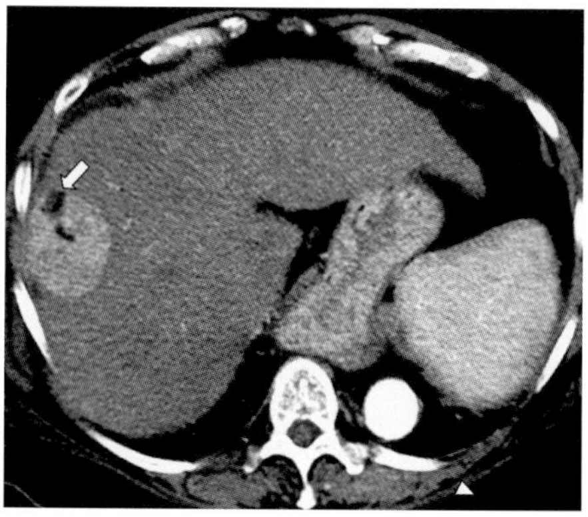

Figure 21.6

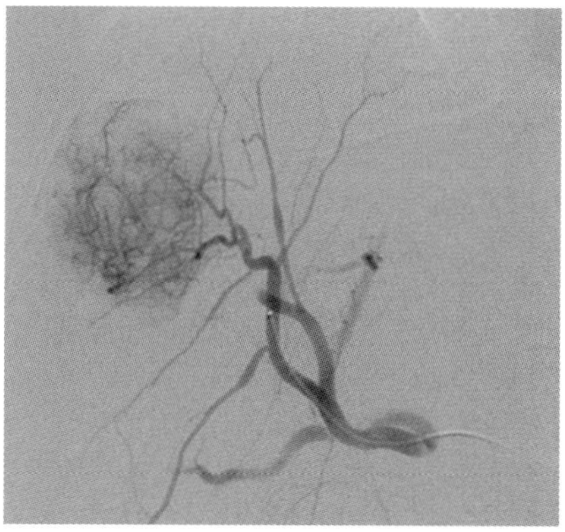

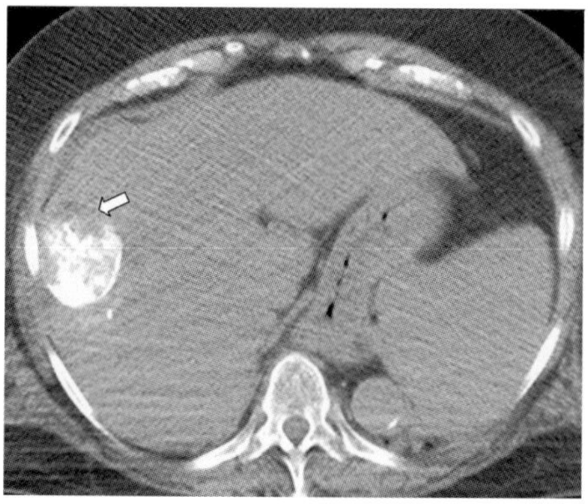

Figure 21.7

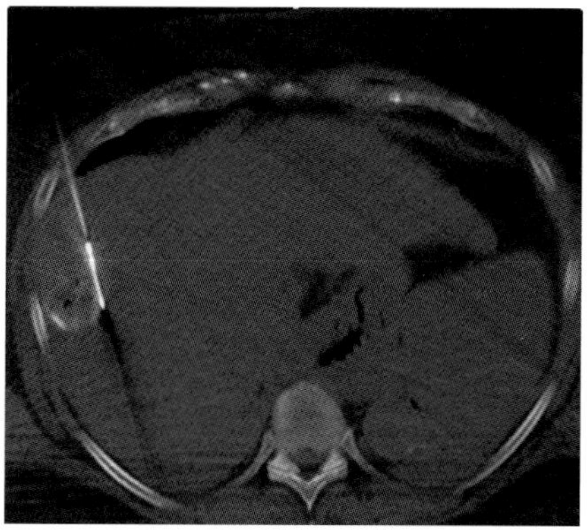

Figure 21.8

Findings

▶ Arterial phase contrast-enhanced computed tomography (CT) shows a hypervascular lesion in a cirrhotic liver (Fig. 21.5). The lesion contains macroscopic fat (arrow), a finding common to hepatocellular carcinoma (HCC) and hepatic adenomata.

▶ Angiography immediately prior to embolization shows the hypervascular tumor corresponding to the findings on CT (Fig. 21.6) Postembolization noncontrast CT (Fig. 21.7) shows contrast retention in the majority of the tumor with a defect in the anterior margin (arrow).

▶ A microwave electrode is seen in the anterior margin of the tumor targeting the area that was suboptimally treated by embolization (Fig. 21.8).

Teaching Points

▶ In a patient with risk factor(s) for HCC, early arterial enhancement with portal venous phase washout in a lesion >1–2 cm is diagnostic of HCC. This is one of few malignancies that may be diagnosed with imaging alone (i.e., does not require tissue confirmation).

▶ Patients with cirrhosis may not be candidates for surgery due to liver dysfunction or nonhepatic comorbidities. Embolization alone is a palliative (i.e., noncurative) procedure. The addition of ablation for appropriate lesions is considered a potentially curative treatment. Ablation alone may be considered for lesions <3 cm; for lesions 3–5 cm, survival following combination of embolization ablation approximates that of surgical resection.

- Extrahepatic supply from branches of the the phrenic, gastroduodenal, superior mesenteric, renal capsular, and/or internal mammary arteries should be considered based on the location of a given lesion. In this case, the phrenic artery was studied but did not demonstrate tumor vascularity.
- Whether bland embolization (as in this case) or chemoembolization with either drug-eluting beads or lipiodol, immediate noncontrast CT after embolization can identify suboptimally treated areas within a tumor. In select cases, these areas may be targeted with ablation.
- Microwave electrodes are bipolar and therefore do not requiregrounding pads. Unlike radiofrequency ablation in which heat is created passively by frictional agitation, microwave provides active heating. This provides a more reliable ablation defect, but it may also be more likely to injure adjacent structures such as bile ducts in the liver or bronchi in the lung leading to bronchopleural fistula in centrally located lung lesions.

Management

- Compared to radiofrequency ablation, microwave ablation results in higher temperatures, faster ablation times, and larger ablation volume. For larger tumors, multiple electrodes can be placed simultaneously.
- When ablation alone is performed, triple-phase CT immediately after ablation may identify untreated areas. Adequate ablation zone should include a margin of 0.5–1 cm.
- Patients with hepatocellular carcinoma have a very high rate of recurrence due to the underlying field defect (parenchymal damage) of cirrhosis and must be followed closely.

Further Reading

Elnekave E, Erinjeri JP, Brown KT, et al. Long-term outcomes comparing surgery to embolization-ablation for treatment of solitary HCC <7 cm. *Ann Surg Oncol*. 2013; *20*(9):2881–2886.

Wang X, Erinjeri JP, Jia X, et al.Pattern of retained contrast on immediate postprocedure computed tomography (CT) after particle embolization of liver tumors predicts subsequent treatment response. *Cardiovasc Intervent Radiol*. 2013; *36*(4):c.

History

▶ A 60-year-old male with metastatic colon cancer status post recent pulmonary metastatectomy is referred to you with the positron emission tomography (PET)/computed tomography (CT) scans shown in Figures 22.1 and 22.2. What are the treatment options for this patient?

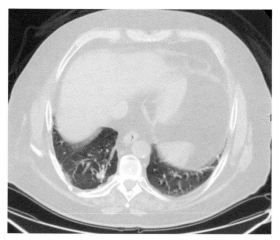

Figure 22.1

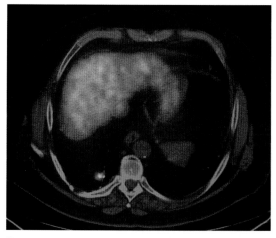

Figure 22.2

Case 22 Lung Ablation

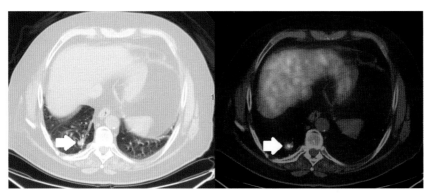

Figure 22.3

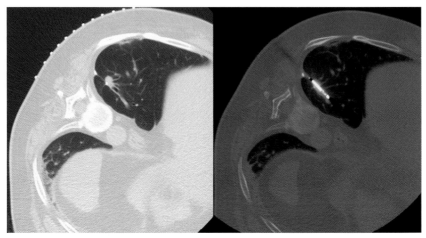

Figure 22.4

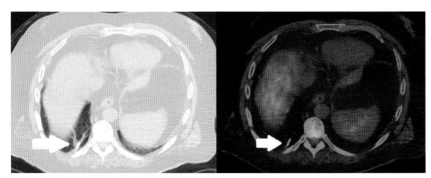

Figure 22.5

Findings

▶ Local tumor recurrence at the staple line (Fig. 22.3, white arrow).

▶ Follow-up PET/CT after pulmonary metastatectomy demonstrates a nodular area of fluorodeoxyglucose (FDG) avidity (arrows) consistent with local tumor recurrence (Fig. 22.3).

- ► Lung ablation was performed Fig. 22.4. Intraprocedural images (left to right) demonstrate the nodule adjacent to the wedge resection site in the right lower lobe followed by an image with a cryoablation probe within the lesion.
- ► A 3-month postablation PET/CT (Fig. 22.5) demonstrates interval decrease in size of the nodule with no residual FDG-avidity (arrows).

Teaching Points

- ► Indications for lung ablation include the following:
  - ■ Early-stage lung cancer in nonsurgical candidates
  - ■ Local tumor recurrence in a previously radiated or postsurgical site
  - ■ Pain palliation in pleural-based disease
- ► Complications include the following:
  - ■ Pneumothorax
  - ■ Hemoptysis (very rarely massive)
  - ■ Broncho-pleural fistula
- ► Similar to considerations with lung biopsy, trajectory should avoid vital structures and limit the number of pleural punctures (see Case 7).
- ► An ablation margin of at least 1.0 cm is recommended to minimize the likelihood of marginal recurrence.
- ► When utilizing microwave or radiofrequency ablative techniques, a ground glass opacity surrounding the target lesion is expected immediately after treatment and corresponds to the ablation zone. With cryoablation, the iceball can be seen as a low-density structure around the cryoprobe.

Management

- ► Most practitioners recommend follow-up imaging (CT or PET/CT) at 3 and 6 months, and every 6 months thereafter.
- ► FDG avidity and ground glass opacity surrounding the target lesion may persist on the 3-month PET/CT, which is used primarily as a baseline for comparison for future scans.
- ► Local tumor recurrence is suspected if new nodular area of FDG avidity is seen not attributable to postablation changes (the latter is typically seen as a thin rim of FDG avidity surrounding the target lesion).
- ► Local tumor recurrences after ablation can and may be retreated with ablation if identified early.

Further Reading

Pua BB, Thornton RH, Solomon SB. Ablation of pulmonary malignancy: current status. *J Vasc Interv Radiol*. 2010; *21*:S223–S232.
Sharma A, Abtin F, Shepard JA. Image-guided ablative therapies for lung cancer. *Radiol Clin North Am*. 2012; *50*:975–999.

History

▶ A 70-Year-Old Female Presents with Hematuria

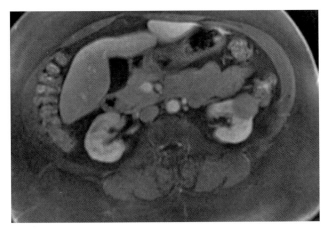

Figure 23.1

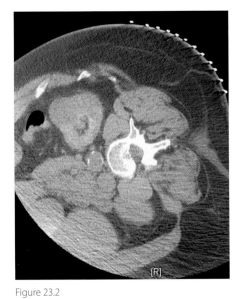

Figure 23.2

Case 23 Renal Cell Carcinoma Treated with Cryoablation

Figure 23.3

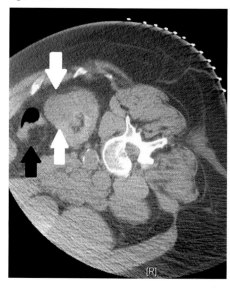

Figure 23.4

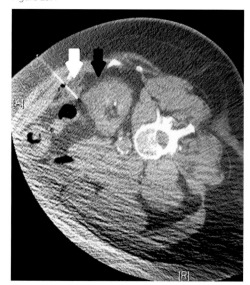

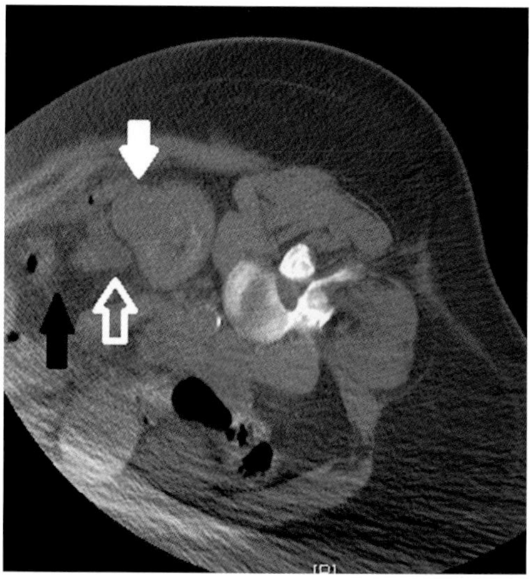

Figure 23.5

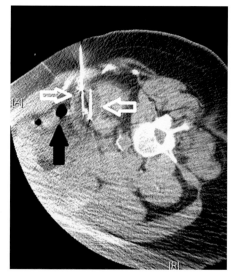

Figure 23.6

Findings

▶ Magnetic resonance imaging (MRI) demonstrates a well-circumscribed lesion within the left kidney demonstrating enhancement pattern suspicious for renal cell carcinoma (Fig. 23.1).

▶ Cryoablation was planned to treat this lesion. However, given the proximity of the lesion (Fig. 23.3, white arrows) to the colon (black arrow), instillation of saline between the colon and renal lesion, was used to separate the two in order to protect the colon from the ablative energy.

▶ A needle (white arrow, Fig. 23.4) has been placed between the colon and renal lesion (black arrow) with gentle saline infusion showing some separation of the two organs.

▶ A more caudal computed tomography (CT) image shows saline (open arrow) creating a potential space between the target lesion (white arrow) and colon (black arrow, Fig. 23.5).

► Figure 23.6 shows two cryoprobes within the lesion with surrounding low density representing the ice ball (open arrows). The black arrow demonstrates air within the colon.

Teaching Points

► Thermal ablation can be performed with heat (microwave/radiofrequency) or cold (cryoablation) energies. Cryoablation allows for visualization of the iceball during the procedure.
► The iceball represents areas where temperatures are <0°C. To achieve satisfactory ablation margins, it should be taken into account that lethal temperature is below –20°C, which occurs 5–6 mm central to the ice ball, depending on the probe manufacturer.
► Short- and long-term outcomes with both radiofrequency ablation and cryoablation show satisfactory overall recurrence free survival when treating small renal masses.
► Most studies suggest that renal function is unaffected by ablative treatment.
► When displacement of an adjacent structure is required in order to perform radiofrequency ablation, sterile water and not saline is used, because the sodium and chloride ions in saline conduct frictional heat to neighboring structures rather than protect them.

Management

► Imaging follow-up is important to promptly identify areas of incomplete ablation or local tumor recurrence allowing for retreatment.
► Cryoablation of central lesions has the potential of damaging the collecting system. Some authors have suggested insertion of a retrograde ureteral catheter to allow for warm saline infusion to protect the collecting system during ablation.

Further Reading

Zagoria RJ, Childs DD. Update on thermal ablation of renal cell carcinoma: oncologic control, technique comparison, renal function preservation, and new modalities. *Curr Urol Rep.* 2012; *13*:63–69.

History

▶ A 68-Year-Old Male with Metastatic Lung Cancer and Hip Pain

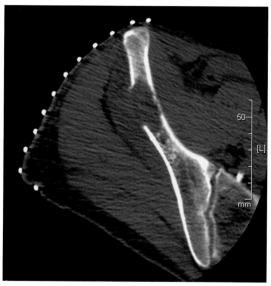

Figure 24.1

Case 24 Cryoablation for Pain Palliation

Figure 24.2

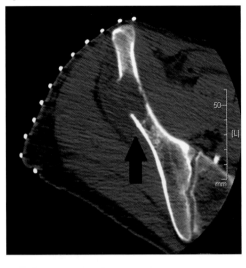

Figure 24.3

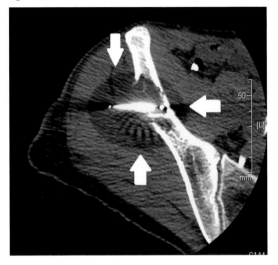

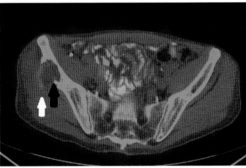

Figure 24.4

Findings

▶ A lytic lesion in seen in the right iliac bone with associated cortical destruction (Fig. 24.3, black arrow).

▶ Two cryoablation probes have been placed within the target lesion with a surrounding low-density ice ball (Fig. 24.4, white arrows) that has formed on both sides of the iliac bone.

▶ Follow-up positron emission tomography (PET)/computed tomography (CT) performed 6 months after ablation (Fig. 24.5) demonstrates no fluorodeoxyglucose (FDG) activity within the lesion (back arrow) and mild activity in the surrounding muscle compatible with postprocedure inflammation (white arrow).

Teaching Points

▶ Cryoablation is performed using specialized probes that provide alternating cycles of active cooling (by expansion of argon gas in a fixed space) and thawing (either passive or active by changing the gas in the probe from argon to helium). This ultimately leads cell death due to rupture of the cell membrane. Typically, two freeze-thaw cycles of 8–10 minutes are used.

▶ When considering ablation as a palliative treatment for painful bone metastases, careful examination of the character, severity, and cause of pain should be considered.

▶ Palliative ablation for pain is indicated in patients with at least moderate pain who have failed oral analgesic therapy and have pain localized to the target lesion.

- Etiology of pain is multifactorial and includes osteoclast-mediated bone remodeling, loss of mechanical strength of affected bone, and activation of adjacent sensory nerve at the bone-tumor intervace.

Management

- Pain control is best achieved by targeting bone-tumor interface. Debulking the tumor mass is a secondary benefit of the procedure.
- The iceball formation can be readily monitored utilizing CT or ultrasound.
- During and immediately after cryoablation for painful bone metastases, patients require less analgesia than patients who undergo radiofrequency ablation.

Further Reading

Kurup AN, Callstrom MR. Ablation of skeletal metastases: current status. *J Vasc Interv Radiol.* 2010; *21*:S242–S250.

History

▶ A 13-Year-Old Girl with a 2 Month History of Left Hip Pain. What is the Best Treatment Option?

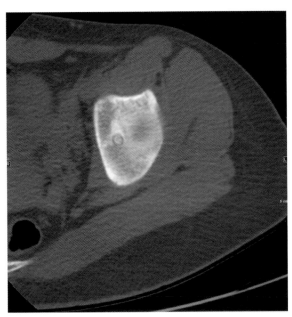

Figure 25.1

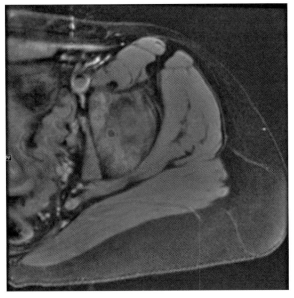

Figure 25.2

Case 25 Osteoid Osteoma

Figure 25.3

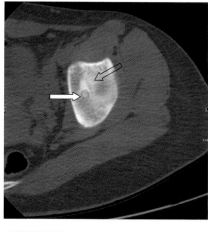

Figure 25.4

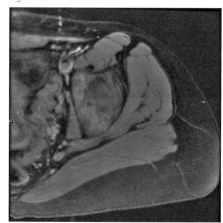

Figure 25.5

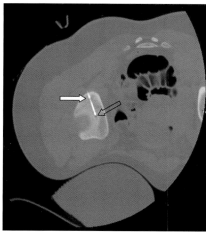

Figure 25.6

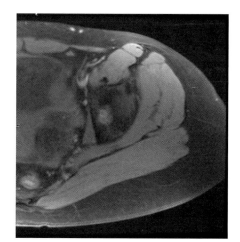

Findings

► On computed tomography (CT), a well-defined nidus (Fig. 25.3, arrow) is seen surrounded by reactive sclerosis (hollow arrow). The nidus is calcified in approximately 50% of patients, as seen in this case.

► On T1-weighted magnetic resonance (MR) (Fig. 25.4), the nidus is isointense to muscle. Peri-nidal inflammation is seen in the surrounding bone marrow.

► Figure 25.5 shows a Cool-tip RF Ablation electrode (Covidien, Mansfield, MA) placed coaxially through the outer cannula of a 15-gauge bone biopsy needle. Note the introducer is just through the cortex (arrow) and approximately 2 cm back from the tip of the electrode (hollow arrow).

► Follow-up image from a T1-weighted MR image 6 weeks after ablation (Fig. 25.6) shows the peri-lesional edema seen on the pretreatment MR (Fig. 25.4) has essentially resolved.

Teaching Points

► Osteoid osteoma is a benign tumor composed of osteoid and woven bone less than 1.5 cm in diameter. They typically occur in juxta-articular bone in young males, most commonly the metaphysis of the femur or tibia.

► The classic history is focal pain, exacerbated at night, and relieved with nonsteroidal anti-inflammatory agents and exercise. Less commonly osteoid osteoma can be a cause of painful scoliosis or bone deformity.

▶ The differential diagnosis includes Brodie's abscess and other rare bone tumors such as intracortical chondroma and osteoblastoma.

Management

▶ Thermal ablation, most commonly radiofrequency ablation, is an attractive minimally invasive treatment option for osteoid osteoma because it is done as an outpatient procedure without minimal recovery time. At the time of the procedure, biopsy is usually performed for pathologic confirmation of the imaging diagnosis.

▶ Radiofrequency ablation of osteoid osteoma is best performed with general anesthesia when possible because the nidus is exquisitely sensitive.

▶ Because of the straight rather than multitined design of the Cool-tip electrode, this is commonly used for ablation of osteoid osteoma. To place the electrode, access to the nidus is achieved with a 15-gauge core biopsy needle, which is used to perform the biopsy prior to advancing the electrode coaxially through the introducer. It is important to ensure that the introducer of the cannula is retracted to at least 1–2 cm back from the tip of the electrode to prevent inadvertent heating of the introducer.

▶ With the Cool-tip electrode, ablation is performed on cautery (not ablation) mode for 6 minutes.

Further Reading

Motamedi D, Learch TJ, Ishimitsu DN, et al. Thermal ablation of osteoid osteoma: overview and step-by-step guide. *Radiographics.* 2009; 29(7):2127–2141.

History

▶ A 67-Year-Old Male with Lung Cancer and a Single, Biopsy-Proven, Adrenal Metastasis

Secondary to cardiopulmonary compromise, he was deemed a poor surgical candidate. The following images illustrate the treatment. However, in the middle of the treatment the patient's blood pressure acutely increases to 200/120 from a baseline of 125/65.

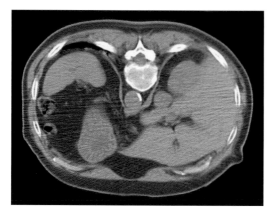

Figure 26.1

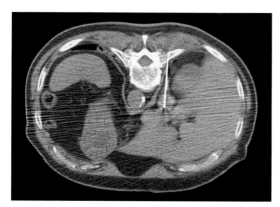

Figure 26.2

Case 26 Hypertensive Crisis during Adrenal Radiofrequency Ablation

Figure 26.3

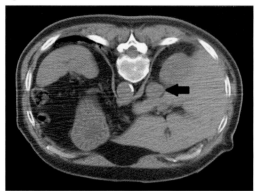

Figure 26.4

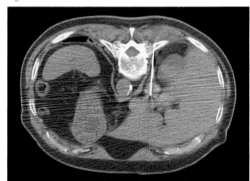

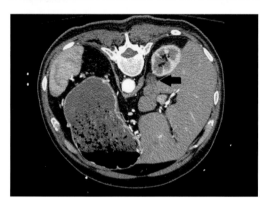

Figure 26.5

Findings

▶ Initial computed tomography (CT) through the level of the adrenal gland demonstrates a nodule (arrow) representing the biopsy-proven adrenal metastasis (Fig. 26.3). Intraprocedural image (Fig. 26.4) demonstrates the ablation probe within the lesion.

▶ Follow-up imaging 29 months after ablation (Fig. 26.5) demonstrates interval decreased size and fullness of the ablated lesion (arrow).

Teaching Points

▶ In nonsurgical candidates, thermal ablation represents a reasonable alternative to treatment of both primary and metastatic adrenal lesions.

▶ During adrenal ablation, acute hypertension is most likely related to systemic catecholamine release by the ablated adrenal tissue.

▶ Because of the concern for catecholamine release during adrenal ablation, some advocate pretreatment with alpha blockade. Oral phenoxybenzamine has been used as pretreatment days to weeks prior to ablation.

▶ Ablation should be performed with constant monitoring of vital signs, especially blood pressure. Hypertensive crisis should be promptly treated by shutting off ablation energy and use of intravenous antihypertensive medication.

  ▪ For RFA and microwave energy, ablation should be shut off.

  ▪ For cryoablation, hypertensive crisis tends to occur during active thaw; rapid refreeze is a potential immediate treatment.

Management

▶ Short-interval office visit after ablation should focus on identification of resolution of clinical syndromes and biochemical markers (for primary adrenal tumors). Antihypertensives should also be adjusted at this time.

▶ Short-interval CT or magnetic resonance imaging (MRI) for a new baseline is performed 1–3 months after ablation and patients are followed with repeat CT or MRI every 3 months to evaluate for local recurrence.

Further Reading

Pua BB, Solomon SB. Ablative therapies for adrenal tumors. *J Surg Oncol.* 2012; *106*:626–631.

Venkatesan AM, Locklin J, Dupuy DE, et al. Percutaneous ablation of adrenal tumors. *Tech Vasc Interv Radiol.* 2010; *13*:89–99.

History

▸ Hepatocellular Carcinoma in a Patient with Hepatitis C Cirrhosis

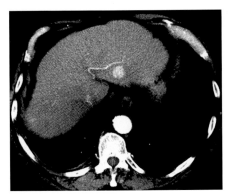

Figure 27.1

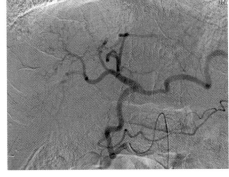

Figure 27.2

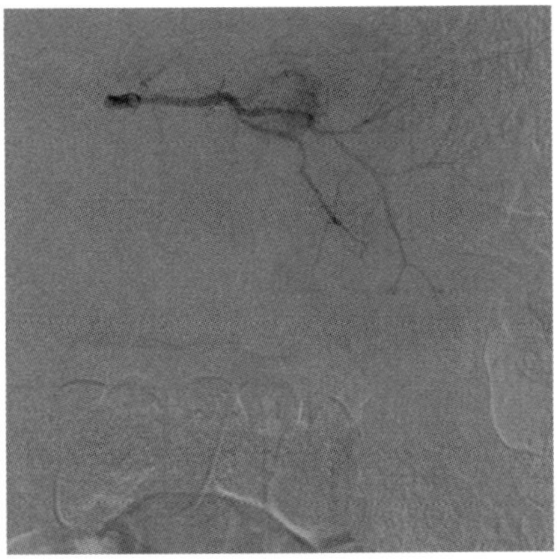

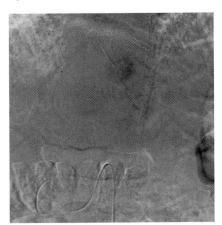

Figure 27.3

Figure 27.4

Case 27 Occluded Celiac Artery with Retrograde Flow through Gastroduodenal Artery

Figure 27.5

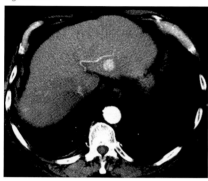

Figure 27.6

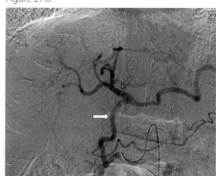

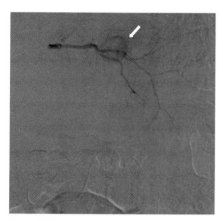

Figure 27.7

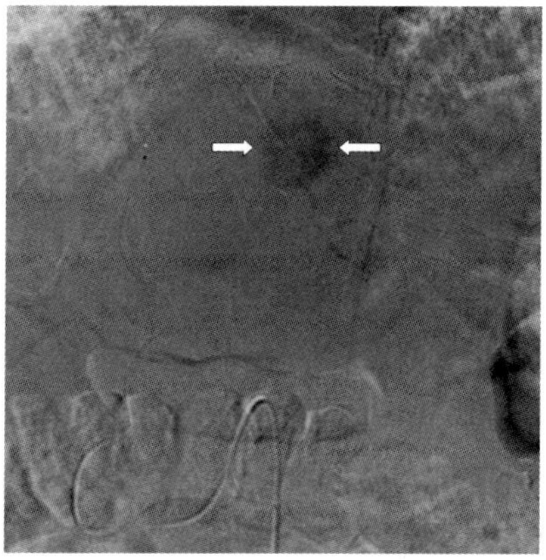

Figure 27.8

Findings

▶ Arterial phase computed tomography (CT) scan of the liver (Fig. 27.5) shows a hypervascular tumor in segment 2. The lobulated contour of the liver is suggestive of cirrhosis.

▶ The inferior pancreaticoduodenal artery arising from the superior mesenteric artery is catheterized with a reverse-curve (Simmons) catheter (Fig. 27.6). Arteriography shows retrograde filling of the gastroduodenal artery (GDA) (arrow) supplying the proper hepatic artery (hollow arrow).

▶ Early-phase (Fig. 27.7) and late-phase (Fig. 27.8) digital subtraction arteriography of the segment 2 hepatic artery shows the tumor blush of the hypervascular mass (arrows) corresponding to the finding on the preprocedural CT scan.

Teaching Points

▶ Classic CT findings of hepatocellular carcinoma include early arterial enhancement with washout on portal venous phase imaging. In patients with risk factors for hepatocellular carcinoma (e.g., cirrhosis, hepatitis B, etc.), the diagnosis is made by imaging findings alone (see Case 21).

▶ Retrograde flow in the GDA is most often associated with either occlusion of the celiac artery or hyperdynamic flow in the hepatic artery due to arteriovenous fistula or extensive hypervascular metastases.

- Collateral circulation between the celiac and superior mesenteric arteries is through the superior and inferior pancreaticoduodenal arcade. The Arc of Buhler is an embryonic remnant connecting the more proximal celiac axis and superior mesenteric artery seen in a small number of patients.

Management

- Prior to undertaking any hepatic intervention, careful review of all imaging is important to identify variant anatomy or other vascular abnormalities (e.g., celiac occlusion) that may impact the procedure.
- In this case, bland hepatic artery embolization (HAE) was performed with 40–120 micron Embospheres ©. Other embolic techniques include transarterial catheter embolization (TACE), embolization with drug-eluting beads (DEBs), and radioembolization (90Y). None has proven superior in overall survival, and each has a slightly different complication profile.
- This patient also had tumors in the right hemi-liver (not shown). Patients with solitary tumors <5 cm or with up to three tumors <3 cm may be eligible for liver transplant under the Milan Criteria. Most patients with cirrhosis are not candidates for surgical resection based on compromised liver function. Only patients with Childs-Pugh A cirrhosis are typically considered for curative resection.
- Patients with hepatocellular carcinoma have a high rate of recurrence due to the underlying field defect of cirrhosis and must be followed closely.

Further Reading

Brown DB, Nikolic B, Covey AM, et al. Quality improvement guidelines for transhepatic arterial chemoembolization, embolization, and chemotherapeutic infusion for hepatic malignancy. *J Vasc Interv Radiol.* 2012; 23(3):287–294

Miyayama S, Matsui O, Taki K, et al. Extrahepatic blood supply to hepatocellular carcinoma: angiographic demonstration and transcatheter arterial chemoembolization. *Cardiovasc Intervent Radiol.* 2006; 29(1):39–48.

History

▶ Fever and Leukocytosis 2 Weeks after Hepatic Artery Embolization

Figure 28.3 is 1 week post embolization and Figure 28.4 is 2 weeks post embolization.

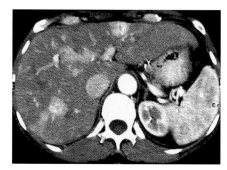

Figure 28.1

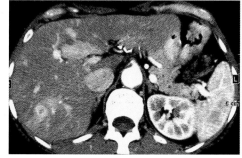

Figure 28.2

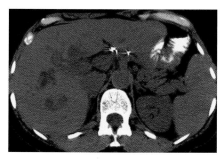

Figure 28.3

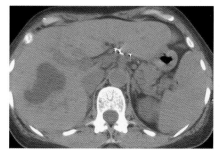

Figure 28.4

Case 28 Liver Abscess after Embolization

Figure 28.5

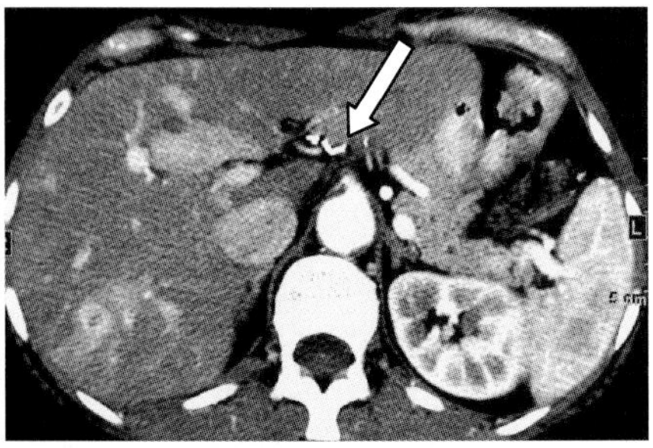

Figure 28.6

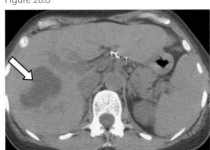

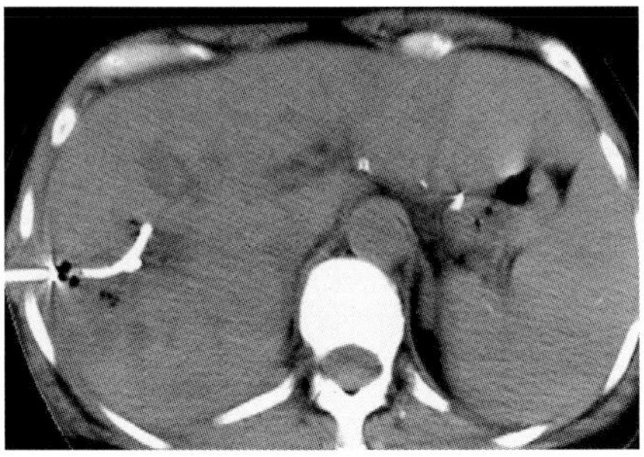

Figure 28.7

Figure 28.8

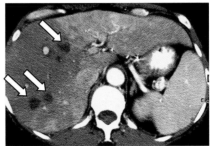

Findings

▶ Multiple hypervascular liver tumors are seen on arterial-phase computed tomography (CT) imaging (Fig. 28.5). Surgical clips (arrow) and an absence of the head and neck of the pancreas on imaging should raise the possibility of prior pancreaticoduodenectomy.

▶ Two weeks after embolization, a low-density collection in the right hemiliver has increased in size compared to both one week earlier and to the tumor seen in that area on the preembolization scan Figures 28.3 and 28.5 respectively (arrow). In the setting of fever and leukocytosis, this is suggestive of an abscess.

▶ Percutaneous abscess drainage was performed (Fig. 28.7). After resolution of the abscess, the low-density lesions in the right liver on 3-month follow-up (Fig. 28.8) represent previously treated necrotic tumors (arrows).

Teaching Points

▶ In the setting of a colonized biliary tree the incidence of postembolization liver abscess is significant— approaching 40% without appropriate antibiotic prophylaxis.

▶ Any procedure that violates the integrity of the sphincter of Oddi results in colonization of the biliary tree. This may be related to prior surgery (e.g., pancreaticoduodenectomy, bilioenteric anastamosis), pappilotomy/ sphincterotomy, or biliary drainage.

▶ Fever and leukocytosis are common following embolization, and the appearance of necrotic tumor secondary to embolization can mimic the appearance of an abscess. One clue that there was an abscess and not simply a treated tumor was that the size of the low-density area was significantly larger than the treated tumor.

▶ Indications for embolization of liver metastases from neuroendocrine tumor include control of hormonal symptoms (e.g., commonly diarrhea, flushing; less common syndromes include hypoglycemia, ACTH production), pain related to tumor bulk, and local tumor control.

Management

▶ Antibiotic prophylaxis for patients with colonized biliary tree should include an antibiotic excreted in the bile, such as piperacillin/tazobactam or cefotetan, and antibiotic prophylaxis should continue several days after the procedure.

Further Reading

Kim W, Clark TW, Baum RA, et al. Risk factors for liver abscess formation after hepatic chemoembolization. *J Vasc Interv Radiol.* 2001; *12*(8):965–968.

History

▶ A 63-Year-Old Female with Rectal Cancer Metastatic to the Liver with Chemotherapy-Resistant Disease

See Figure 29.1. What treatment is this patient being prepared for?

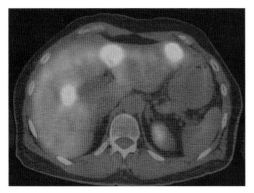

Figure 29.1

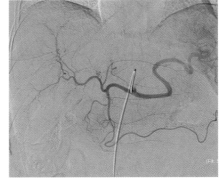

Figure 29.2

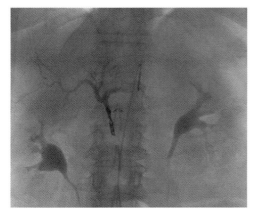

Figure 29.3

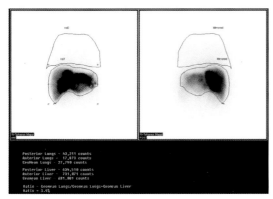

Figure 29.4

Case 29 Transarterial Embolization with Y-90

Figure 29.5

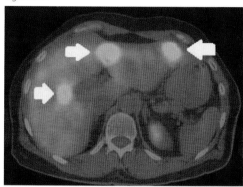

Figure 29.6

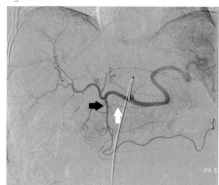

Figure 29.7

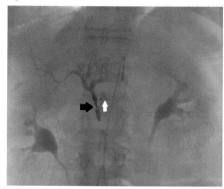

Figure 29.8

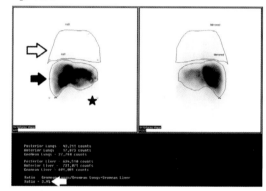

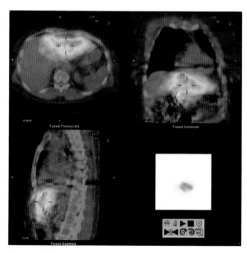

Figure 29.9

Findings

▶ Figure 29.5 demonstrates fluorodeoxyglucose (FDG)-avid metastatic disease in both the right and left hemilivers (white arrows).

▶ Figure 29.6 is a digital subtraction angiogram from an anatomic mapping procedure prior to Yittrium-90 (Y-90) therapy administered on a subsequent visit. The gastroduodenal artery (black arrow) and right gastric artery (white arrow) are visualized in this celiac arteriogram. These vessels are subsequently coil embolized as seen on Figure 29.7.

▶ ^{99m}Tc-labeled MAA is injected from the proper hepatic artery, and the patient was sent for a gamma emission count as shown in Figure 29.8. A shunt fraction of 3.9% (white arrow) was identified. It is important to review the emission scan for homogenous emission in the liver (solid black arrow), to confirm minimal lung emission (hollow black arrow), and to confirm absence of uptake in the stomach and small bowel (star).

▶ After a proper Y-90 dose is calculated, the patient returns for a second procedure for Y-90 treatment of the left hemiliver. Figure 29.9 shows the follow-up Bremsstrahlung scan confirming treatment confined to the left hemiliver.

Teaching Points

▶ Y-90 is created by bombardment of yttrium-89 with neutrons in a reactor. Y-90 is unstable (half-life: 2.67 days) and decays to zirconium-90, releasing a beta particle. This beta particle has a penetrance of 2.5–11 mm in tissue and is the basis of delivering radiotherapy to the target tumor.

▶ Y-90 treatment refers to transarterial delivery of this radioactive element to the target tumor by coupling it with a microsphere delivery device, whether via a glass microsphere (TheraSphere; MDS Nordion, Ottawa, Ontario, Canada) or plastic resin microsphere (SIR-Spheres; Sirtex Medical, Sydney, Australia).

▶ There are two absolute contraindications for transarterial Y-90 therapy: uncontrolled reflux into arteries feeding the gastroduodenal region and excessive shunting to the lungs. Meticulous mapping is of utmost importance:

  ▪ The superior mesenteric artery, and celiac and hepatic arterial branches are evaluated, and embolization of the gastroduodenal artery, right gastric artery, and any other accessory arteries to prevent reflux into the gastrointestinal system should be considered and/or performed.

  ▪ With the microcatheter in the hepatic arterial branch to be treated, scintigraphy with the injection of 4–6 mCi of ^{99m}Tc-labeled MAA is performed. Hepatopulmonary shunt fraction is calculated as a ratio of the gamma emission count in the lung to that of liver.

  ▪ Y-90 microsphere embolization should not be performed in patients with (1) shunt fraction indicating radiation exposure to the lungs to exceed 30Gy, (2) shunt fraction greater than 20% of the injected dose, or (3) in the setting of uncorrectable (by coil embolization) flow to the gastrointestinal organs.

▶ The prescribed dose of Y-90, or written directive, includes the total radiation dose to be administered to the liver, the form of the Y-90 microspheres, and the maximum acceptable dose at extrahepatic sites where there may be shunting.

  ▪ Radiation dose calculation differs depending on microspheres used (glass or resin).

Management

▶ A single-photon emission computed tomography (SPECT)/computed tomography (CT) Bremsstrahlung scan can be performed within 30 hours after infusion therapy to confirm distribution of Y-90 in the liver as well as to detect any extrahepatic distribution.

▶ After Y-90 therapy, a CT scan of the treated liver will demonstrate low attenuation in the treatment region. These areas of low attenuation may be heterogeneous, especially when a relatively low absorbed dose of radiation is utilized. Care should be taken to not misinterpret this as recurrence.

▶ For patients with bilobar disease, treating each hemiliver on separate occasions may decrease hepatic toxicity.

Further Reading

Murthy R, Nunez R, Szklaruk F, et al. Yttrium-90 microsphere therapy for hepatic malignancy: devices, indications, technical considerations, and potential complications. *Radiographics*. 2005; 25:S41–S55.

► Incidental Finding on Preoperative Computed Tomography Scan. What is the Appropriate Management of this Finding?

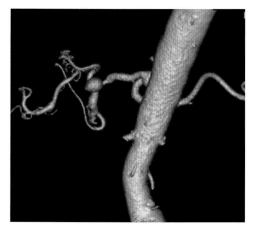

Figure 30.1

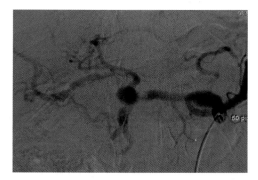

Figure 30.2

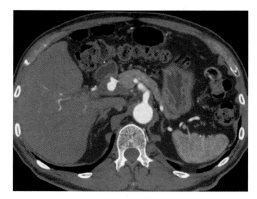

Figure 30.3

Case 30 Hepatic Artery Aneurysm

Figure 30.4

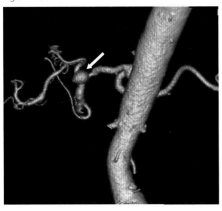

Figure 30.5

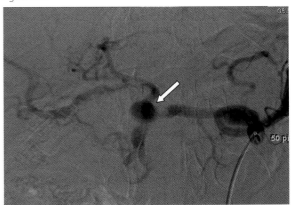

Figure 30.6

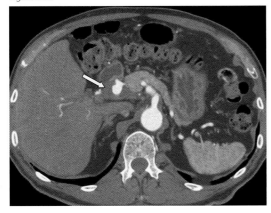

Figure 30.7

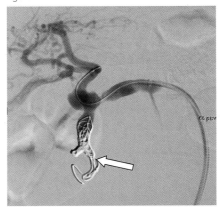

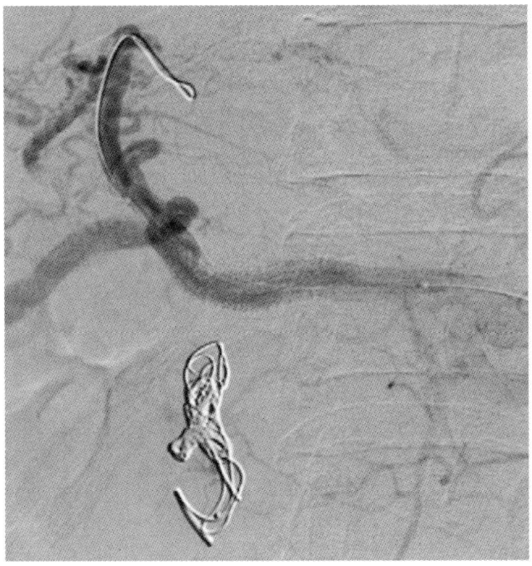

Figure 30.8

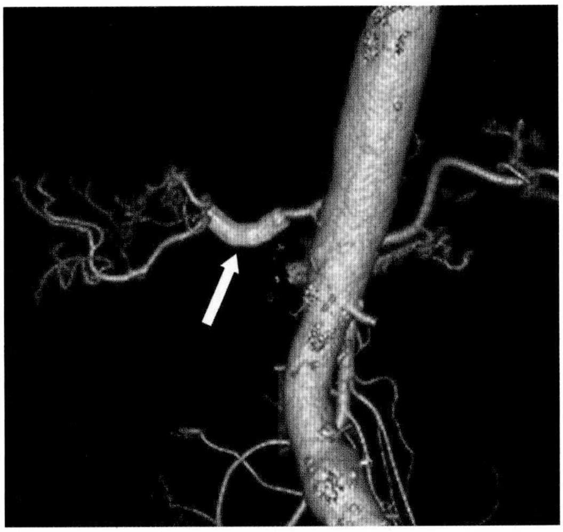

Figure 30.9

Findings

▶ Reconstruction from an arterial-phase computed tomography (CT) scan (Fig. 30.4) and a single image from a digital subtraction angiogram (Fig. 30.5) demonstrate a saccular aneurysm (arrow) of the common hepatic artery at the bifurcation into the proper hepatic and gastroduodenal arteries. A single axial image shows this to be partially thrombosed (Fig. 30.6, arrow).

▶ Figure 30.7 shows a common hepatic angiogram after embolization of the gastroduodenal artery, which was done to prevent retrograde flow from the superior mesenteric artery from causing an endoleak (arrow).

▶ After placement of a stent-graft extending from the common hepatic artery into the proper hepatic artery just proximal to the bifurcation into right and left hepatic arteries (Fig. 30.8), there is no further filling of the aneurysm sac.

▶ One month later, reconstruction from an arterial-phase CT (Fig. 30.9) shows the covered stent in good position with no filling of the aneurysm sac or the embolized gastroduodenal artery.

Teaching Points

▶ True aneurysms represent saccular or fusiform dilation of a vessel whose wall is intact (i.e., all three layers of the vessel wall are present in the aneurysm). This is in contradistinction from pseudoaneurysms (which are much more common) that can be thought of as contained rupture with loss of the integrity of at least one layer of the vessel wall. Most pseudoaneurysms require treatment, whereas true aneurysms are treated based on size or interval growth in order to prevent rupture.

▶ The most common visceral artery aneurysms involve the splenic artery.

▶ Hepatic artery aneurysms can be associated with celiac artery stenosis and the presence of a median arcuate ligament.

▶ Indications for treatment include symptomatic aneurysms (e.g., pain), size >2 cm, or rapid growth.

Management

▶ Both pseudoaneurysms and true aneurysms may be treated successfully with stent-graft placement across the lesion. True aneurysms may be obliterated by filling the aneurysm sac with coils, onyx, or glue. Pseudoaneurysms, on the other hand, because they are contained ruptures, require occlusion of the vessel immediately proximal and distal to the injury. An exception is catheter-related femoral artery pseudoaneurysms, which have been successfully treated with thrombin injection.

▶ The size of visceral stent-grafts can be determined by measuring the diameter of the vessel proximal to the aneurysm where the walls are parallel and oversizing by 10%–20%.

▶ If a stent-graft cannot be placed to treat a hepatic artery aneurysm, embolization of the hepatic artery proximal and distal to the aneurysm is a reasonable alternative in the setting of a patent portal vein.

▶ After placement of a visceral artery stent-graft, consideration of short-term antiplatelet therapy should be considered.

Further Reading

Jackson, James E. Management of Visceral Aneurysms in Image guided interventions. Mauro, M, Murphy K, Thomson K, Venbrux A, Morgan R editors. Philadelphia, PA: Elsevier Saunders, 2013:508–515.

History

▶ Renal Cell Carcinoma Status Post Fall

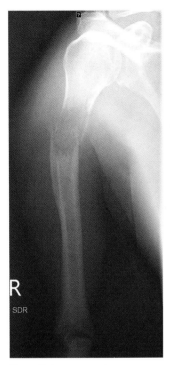

Figure 31.1

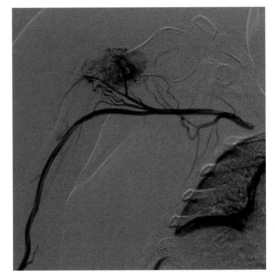

Figure 31.2

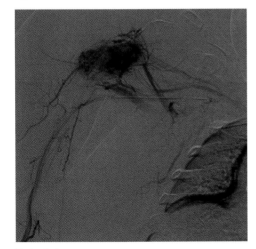

Figure 31.3

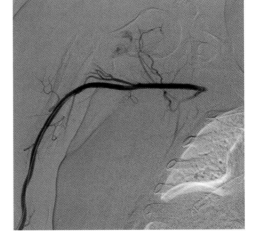

Figure 31.4

Case 31   Embolization of Renal Cell Carcinoma Bone Metastasis

Figure 31.5

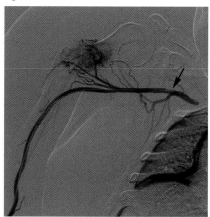

Figure 31.6

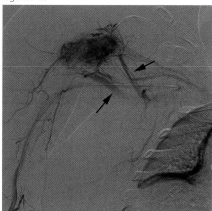

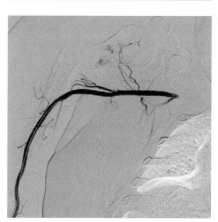

Figure 31.7

Findings

- ▶ Radiograph of the right humerus (Fig. 31.1) shows a displaced fracture of the proximal diaphysis at the site of a lytic metastasis.
- ▶ An angiographic catheter has been placed from right radial artery approach into the right subclavian artery. Note catheter tip (Fig. 31.5, arrow) and catheter course in Figure 31.6.
- ▶ At the fracture site, a hypervascular soft tissue mass is identified (Fig. 31.6). Draining veins are seen coursing medially from the tumor (arrows).
- ▶ After embolization (Fig. 31.7) the mass is markedly less vascular. The subclavian artery remains widely patent.

Teaching Points

- ▶ Radial access may be performed safely after confirmation of a patent palmar arch in the hand using the Allen test. Radial artery access was chosen in this case to avoid the risk of stroke from catheter manipulation in the aortic arch across the origins of the carotid arteries.
- ▶ Preoperative embolization of hypervascular tumors has been shown to reduce intraoperative blood loss and transfusion requirement. The most common hypervascular bone metastases include renal cell carcinoma, as in this case, multiple myeloma and thyroid carcinoma.

▶ It is important to determine whether early visualization of draining veins represents a shunt, because embolization in this setting would result in nontarget embolization to the lungs. When in doubt, use of larger particles or PVA, which tends to clump and result in a slightly more proximal embolization, should be considered.

Management

▶ After preoperative bone embolization, surgery should be performed within 3 days to minimize revascularization of the tumor from collateral vessels.

▶ On occasion, embolization of a spine tumor may be performed in the absence of planned surgery to prevent neural encroachment.

Further Reading

Owen RJT. Embolization of musculoskeletal bone tumors. *Semin Intervent Radiol.* 2010; 27(2):111–123.

History

▶ An 85-Year-Old Male with Massive Hemoptysis

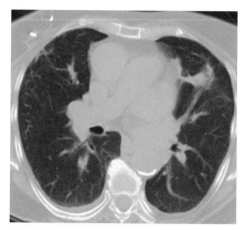

Figure 32.1

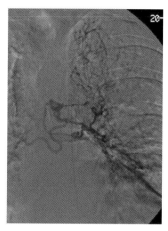
Figure 32.2

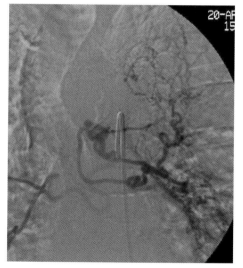
Figure 32.3

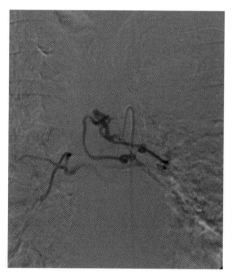
Figure 32.4

Case 32   Bronchial Artery Embolization

Figure 32.5

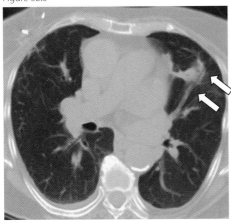

Figure 32.6

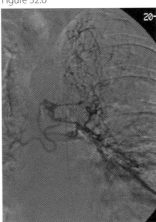

Figure 32.7

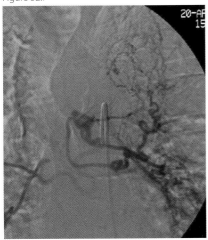

Figure 32.8

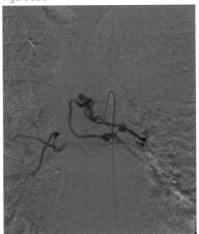

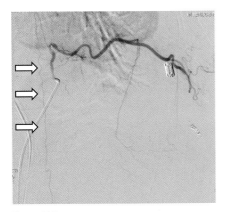

Figure 32.9

Findings

▶ Single image from a computed tomography (CT) (Fig. 32.5) shows bronchiectasis and air space disease in the lingula (arrows).

▶ Bronchial artery angiogram (Figs. 32.6 and 32.7) demonstrates a markedly hypertrophied left bronchial artery. No active extravasation is seen.

▶ Immediately after embolization with large particles, there is no longer fillling of the bronchial artery branches (Fig. 32.8).

▶ In another patient (Fig. 32.9), an intercostal angiogram demonstrates an accessory anterior spinal artery (arrows), which can also arise from the bronchial artery.

Teaching Points

▶ Bronchial arteries most commonly arise from the descending thoracic aorta between T4 and T8. The most common configuration is a single right and multiple left arteries, although this is quite variable. Other potential sites of origin include internal mammary, subclavian, thyrocervical, phrenic, and intercostal arteries.

▶ Common causes of hemoptysis requiring intervention include chronic inflammatory conditions such as cystic fibrosis, tuberculosis, aspergillosis, bronchiectasis, and, as in this case, malignancy.

▶ The anterior spinal artery may have medullary branches arising from proximal bronchial arteries. Embolization of the anterior spinal artery can cause permanent paralysis and must be avoided. The charateristic "hairpin" loop (Fig. 32.9) and consistent position over the spine in multiple obliquities are clues to the presence of a spinal artery branch.

Management

▶ The definition of massive hemoptysis varies, ranging from 200 to 600 cc/day. Treatment is generally indicated to prevent/minimize the risk of aspiration and asphyxiation.

▶ It is rare to see active extravasation from the bronchial arteries. Most patients with massive hemoptysis have diffuse lung disease and hence diffusely abnormal bronchial arteries. For that reason, lateralization of hemoptysis before embolization using bronchoscopy is very helpful in preprocedure planning.

▶ Although a less common cause of hemoptysis, bleeding from a pulmonary artery source should also be considered when hemoptysis is not controlled with bronchial artery embolization or a structural abnormality of the pulmonary artery is detected by CT.

▶ Immediate success rate is approximately 85%; however, recurrent hemoptysis is relatively common due to recanalization or hypertrophy of collateral vessels or due to progression of the underlying process. Embolization with particles (rather than coils) is recommended as coil embolizaiton makes subsequent intervention more complicated.

Further Reading

Bronchial artery embolization. In: Mauro, Murphy, Thomson, Venbruz, and Zollikofer, eds.: *Image-Guided Interventions*, volume 2. Philadelphia, PA: Saunders Elsevier, 2008:931–938.

History

▶ A 54-year-old woman was referred from a pulmonologist after she presented with progressive shortness of breath. The patient has an abnormal echocardiographic bubble study and the following findings. What is the appropriate management?

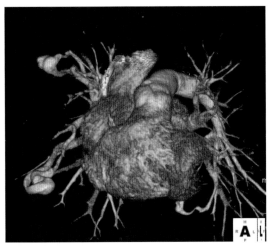

Figure 33.1

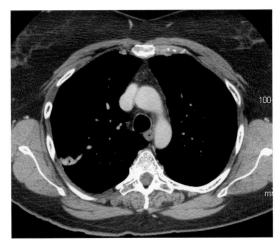

Figure 33.2

Case 33   Pulmonary Arteriovenous Malformation

Figure 33.3

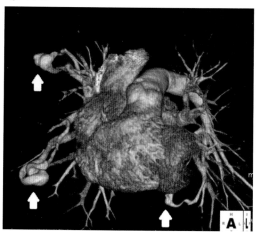

Figure 33.4

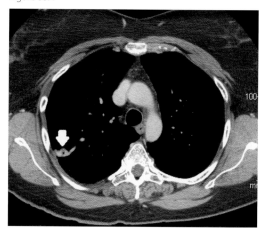

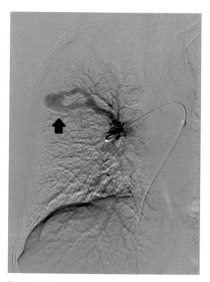

Figure 33.5

Figure 33.6

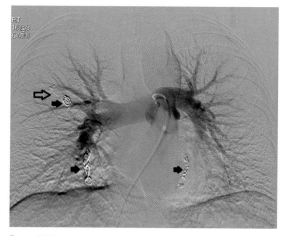

Findings

▶ Contrast-enhanced computed tomography (CT) angiogram (Fig. 33.4) and three-dimensional reconstruction (Fig. 33.3) demonstrate three simple pulmonary arteriovenous malformations (arrows) as characterized by a single feeding artery entering the aneurysmal segment followed by a draining vein. Malformations are identified in the right middle and lower lobes as well as the left lower lobe.

▶ Figure 33.5 is a digital subtraction angiogram (DSA) with a catheter in the distal right main pulmonary artery. The pulmonary arteriovenous malformation (PAVM) in the right middle lobe (arrow) is shown. The PAVM within the right lower lobe does not become evident until after embolization of the PAVM within the right middle lobe due to the large shunt from this malformation.

▶ DSA image with a flush catheter in the main pulmonary artery (Fig. 33.6) following successful embolization of all three PAVMs. An amplatzer vascular occlusion device (hollow arrow) was used in the PAVM within the right middle lobe in addition to metallic coils due to its size. The remaining PAVMs were embolized utilizing metallic coils (arrows).

Teaching Points

▶ Presenting symptoms may include hypoxia, transient ischemic attacks, stroke, cerebral abscess, and/or hemoptysis.

▶ If left untreated, Gossage et al. (1998) calculated stroke incidence to be 11.4%, brain abscess 6.8% with total morbidity, and mortality at 23%.

▶ Traditional teaching suggests that all detected AVMs with feeding arteries larger than 3 mm in adults should be treated; some authors have suggested treatment of any detected PAVMs.

▶ Between 60% and 90% of patients with PAVMs have hereditary hemorrhagic telangiectasia (HHT).

▶ Catheter and wire exchanges should be performed in a saline bath to diminish the risk of paradoxical air emboli.

Management

▶ Patients with suspected HHT should have family members screened for the disease with genetic testing. Family members should also be screened with an echocardiographic bubble study.

▶ Between 10% and 20% of patients with HHT will have cerebral vascular malformations, and magnetic resonance imaging (MRI) should be performed for evaluation. Other manifestations of HHT include visceral telangectasias such as in the gastrointestinal tract and liver. These are treated symptomatically and routine screening is not recommended.

▶ Following embolization of a PAVM in a patient with HHT, follow up with contrast chest CT scans, or to minimize radiation exposure, echocardiographic bubble study is recommended.

Further Reading

Faughnan ME, Palda VA, Garcia-Tsao G, et al. International guidelines for the diagnosis and management of hereditary haemorrhagic telangiectasia. *J Med Genet*. 2011; 48:73–87.

Gossage JR, Kanj G. Pulmonary arteriovenous malformations. A state of the art review. *Am J Respir Crit Care Med*. 1998; 158:643–661.

Meek ME, Meek JC, Beheshti MV. Management of pulmonary arteriovenous malformations. *Semin Intervent Radiol*. 2011; 28:24–31.

History

▶ A 45-Year-Old Female with Persistent, Disabling Pelvic Fullness

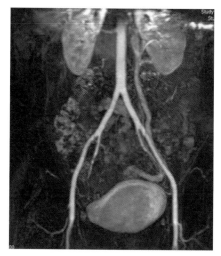

Figure 34.1

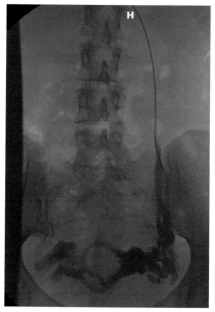

Figure 34.2

Case 34 Pelvic Congestion Syndrome

Figure 34.3

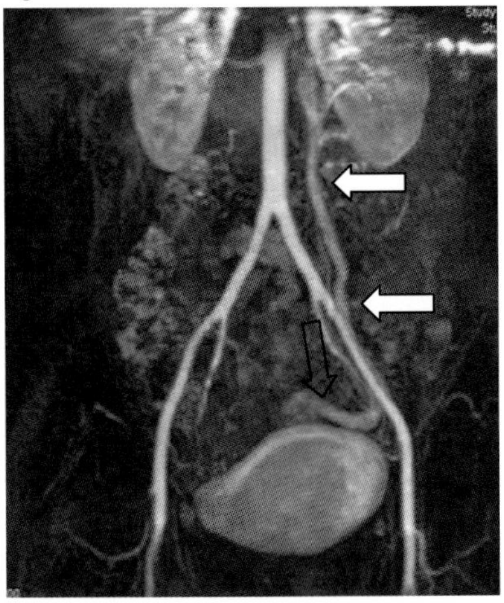

Figure 34.4

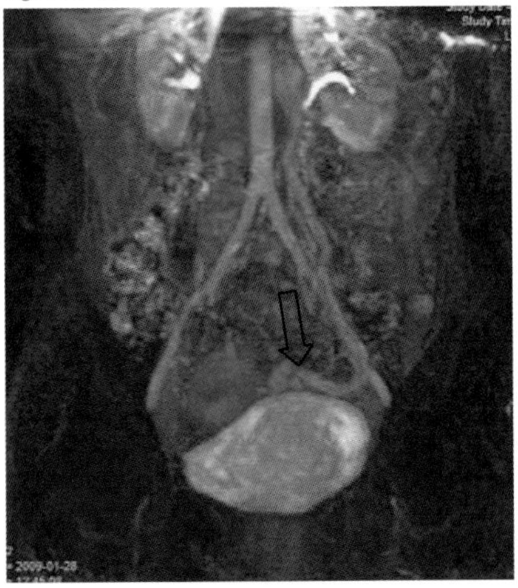

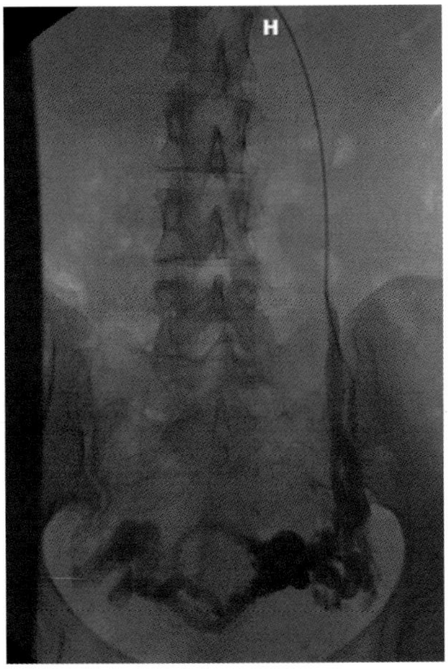

Figure 34.5

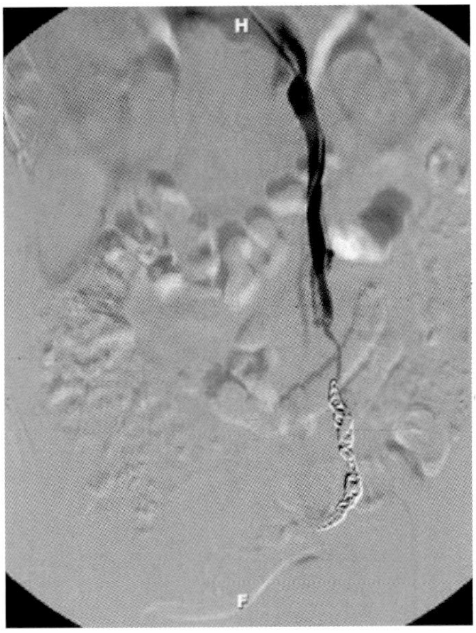

Figure 34.6

Findings

▶ Coronal magnetic resonance (MR) images demonstrate an enlarged ovarian vein draining pelvic varices (Figs. 34.3 and 34.4, arrows).

▶ The left ovarian vein has been catheterized via the left renal vein (Fig. 34.5). Venography confirms the MR findings of engorged pelvic veins. Note the more distal veins should be smaller in caliber than the vein into which they drain.

▶ After embolization with sodium tetradecyl sulfate and coils, there is no residual filling of the pelvic variscosities (Fig. 34.6).

Teaching Points

▶ Incompetence of valves and retrograde flow in an engorged ovarian vein can manifest as chronic pelvic pain, which is defined as noncyclic pelvic pain for at least 6 months. This constellation is known as "pelvic congestion syndrome." Hemodynamically, this is analogous to the male varicocele (see Case 42).

▶ Pelvic congestion syndrome usually presents in premenopausal women as unilateral pelvic pain exacerbated with standing, lifting, and sexual intercourse.

▶ The differential diagnosis of chronic pelvic pain in women is broad, and it includes endometriosis, fibroids, adhesions from pelvic inflammatory disease, atypical menstrual pain, urologic disorders, and inflammatory bowel disease. Pelvic inflammatory disease should be ruled out prior to consideration of embolization. In some patients, vulvar varicosities can be seen involving the upper medial thigh.

▶ Noninvasive imaging is often performed early in the initial workup of pelvic congestion syndrome, and it is particularly useful in excluding other etiologies. Ovarian vein diameter >5 mm with slow flow and/or dilated pelvic veins suggest the diagnosis, but catheter venography remains the gold standard. Findings at venography suggestive of the syndrome include ovarian vein reflux with incompetent valves and contrast filling vessels across the midline.

Management

▶ Treatment options include surgical ligation of the ovarian veins, hysterectomy, and transcatheter embolization.

▶ Venography while the patient is performing a Valsalva maneuver is helpful to confirm the presence of incompetent valves with reflux into pelvic varicosities. Ideally, this would be performed in a semierect position, but in practice this is difficult to accomplish.

▶ Similar to internal spermatic vein embolization for varicocele, treatment includes embolization of the offending vein. This can be accomplished with coil embolization, foamed sodium tetradecyl sulfate, n-butyl cyanoacrylate, or the Amplatzer device.

▶ Embolization should start at the level of the sciatic notch and progress cranial to within a few centimeters from the insertion of the ovarian vein into the inferior vena cava (right) or renal vein (left).

▶ Bilateral ovarian vein embolization is often performed. This is in contradistinction to internal spermatic vein embolization in which embolization is often only performed on the side of the varicocele.

▶ Significant improvement in pelvic pain is seen in 70%–80% following embolization, with a recurrence of symptoms in 5% over time. There is no evidence of alteration of menstrual cycle or fertility.

▶ In patients with persistent symptoms after embolization, interrogation and embolization of varices seen arising from the anterior division of the internal iliac veins may be considered.

Further Reading

Bittles MA, Hoffer EK. Gonadal vein embolization: treatment of varicocele and pelvic congestion syndrome. *Semin Intervent Radiol.* 2008; 25(3):261–70.

Katz MD, Sugay SB, Walker DK, Palmer SL, Marx MV. Beyond hemostasis: spectrum of gynecologic and obstetric indications for transcatheter embolization. *Radiographics.* 2012; 32(6):1713–31. doi: 10.1148/rg.326125524.

▶ A 45-Year-Old Female with Acute Right-Sided Flank Pain

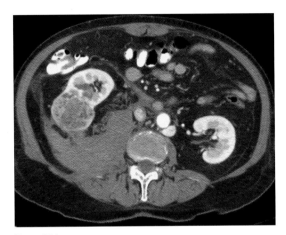

Figure 35.1

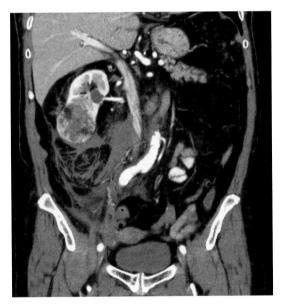

Figure 35.2

Case 35 Ruptured Renal Angiomyolipoma

Figure 35.3

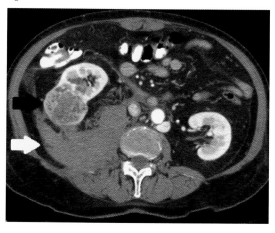

Figure 35.4

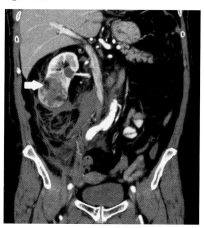

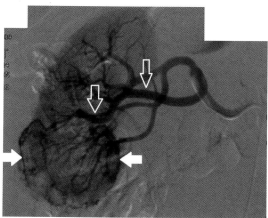

Figure 35.5

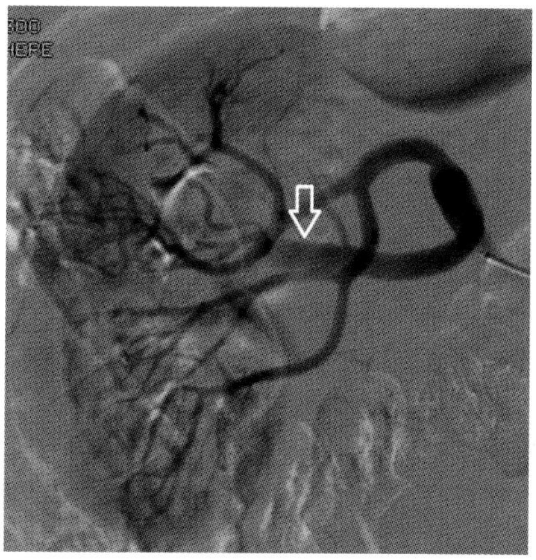

Figure 35.6

Findings

▶ An exophytic lesion (Fig. 35.3, black arrow) is shown arising from the lower pole of the right kidney with associated high-density material in the retroperitoneum representing hemorrhage (white arrow).

▶ Coronal computed tomography (CT) image through the same region (Fig. 35.4) exemplifies fat density material within the lesion (white arrow), confirming the diagnosis of a ruptured angiomyolipoma (AML).

▶ Right renal arteriogram (Fig. 35.5) demonstrates filling of the tumor with associated tortuous tumor vasculature (white solid arrows). Of note, superselective angiogram of one of these segmental renal arteries (white hollow arrow) reveals that most of the supply of this tumor is from this artery.

▶ Renal arteriogram after particle embolization of the segmental artery supplying the tumor (white hollow arrow) with contrast stasis in the stump and no distal flow. Tumor vasculature is no longer seen.

Teaching Points

▶ Renal AML is the most common benign renal neoplasm.

▶ Treatment is reserved for patients with hemorrhage, pain, or for tumors larger than 4 cm because they are at high risk of hemorrhage.

▶ Active contrast extravasation in the setting of acute hemorrhage may not always be identified on angiography, as the surrounding hematoma may obscure the bleeding.

- There is no consensus as to the embolic material of choice.
- Multiple AMLs may be seen in the setting of tuberous sclerosis.

Management
- Follow-up imaging should demonstrate cessation of bleeding with reduction of hematoma.
- After embolization, follow-up imaging should show the tumor to decrease in size; however, the fatty component of AMLs are relatively insensitive to embolization, and therefore there is variability in size reduction.
- Lifelong follow-up is suggested in patients with associated tuberous sclerosis complex secondary to high tumor recurrence rates.

Further Reading
Han YM, Kim JK, Roh BS, et al. Renal angiomyolipoma: selective arterial embolization—effectiveness and changes in angiomyogenic components in long term follow-up. *Radiology*. 1997; 204:65–70.

Kothary N, Soulen MC, Clark TW, et al. Renal angiomyolipoma: long-term results after arterial embolization. *J Vasc Interv Radiol*. 2005; 16:45–50.

History

▶ A 12-Year-Old Girl Kicked by a Horse. What are the Treatment Options?

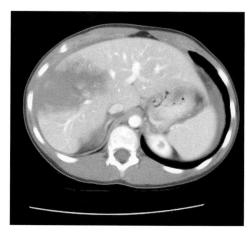

Figure 36.1

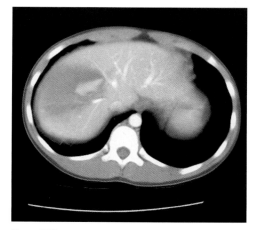

Figure 36.2

Case 36 Liver Trauma

Figure 36.3

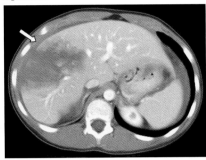

Figure 36.4

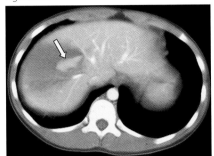

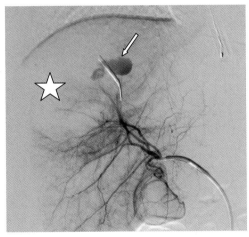

Figure 36.5

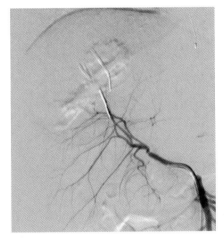

Figure 36.6

Findings

▶ Two images from a contrast-enhanced computed tomography (CT) (Figs. 36.3 and 36.4) show a liver parenchyma fracture with a small subcapsular hematoma (arrow, Fig. 36.3) and active extravasation of contrast (arrow, Fig. 36.4).

▶ Hepatic artery angiogram shows active extravasation from a branch of the right hepatic artery (Fig. 36.5, arrow, after placement of a single straight coil) corresponding to the finding on CT. Also note relative hypoperfusion of the liver supplied by this branch of the hepatic artery (star) and the mass effect crowding branches of the more caudal right hepatic artery.

▶ After embolization with additional straight coils (Fig. 36.6), extravasation is no longer seen.

Teaching Points

▶ The liver is the second most commonly injured intraabdominal organ in blunt trauma and penetrating trauma.

▶ To facilitate communication between radiologists and surgeons and to help guide treatment, grades of liver injury have been developed. This case represents a grade IV injury.

    Grade I—subcapsular hematoma <10% surface area, or capsular tear <1 cm of parenchymal depth

    Grade II—subcapsular hematoma 10%–50% of surface area, or laceration 1–3 cm deep and <10 cm long

    Grade III—subcapsular hematoma >50% surface area, or laceration >3 cm of parenchymal depth

    Grade IV—parenchymal disruption 24%–75% of single lobe or 1–3 Couinaud segments in a single lobe

Grade V—parenchymal disruption >75% of single lobe or >3 Couinaud segments in a single lobe, juxtahepatic venous injury (hepatic vein, inferior vena cava)

Grade VI—hepatic avulsion

► Because the liver parenchyma derives up to 80% of nutrient blood supply from the portal vein, in the setting of a patent portal vein, embolization of the entire hepatic artery rarely causes permanent liver damage.

Management

► Hemodynamic, instability and peritonitis after abdominal trauma are indications for urgent laparotomy. Stable patients should have a contrast-enhanced CT. Hepatic angiography and embolization should be considered as a first-line treatment of (1) patients with transient response to resuscitation, (2) in hemodynamically stable patients with evidence of active extravasation on CT, and (3) hemodynamically stable patients who rebleed after surgical intervention.

► Most patients with liver laceration are managed conservatively, with fewer than 1 in 5 requiring surgical intervention.

Further Reading

The American Association for the Surgery of Trauma Injury Scoring Scale. http://www.aast.org/library/traumatools/injuryscoringscales.aspx. Accessed November 10, 2013.

Malhotra AK, Fabian TC, Croce MA, et al. Blunt hepatic injury: a paradigm shift from operative to nonoperative management in the 1990s. *Ann Surg.* 2000; 231:804.

Ong CC, Toh L, Lo RH, et al. Primary hepatic artery embolization in pediatric blunt hepatic trauma. *J Pediatr Surg.* 2012; 47(12):2316–2320.

Stassen N, Bhullar I, et al. Nonoperative management of blunt hepatic injury: An Eastern Association for the Surgery of Trauma practice management guideline. *J Trauma Acute Care Surg.* 2012; 73:S288.

History

▶ A 14-Year-Old Girl with Left Upper Quadrant Pain Following a Motor Vehicle Accident

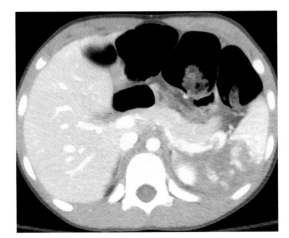

Figure 37.1

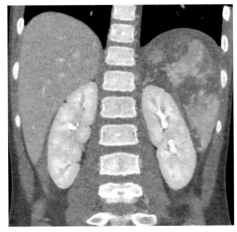

Figure 37.2

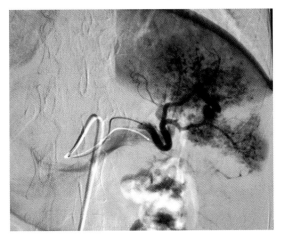

Figure 37.3

Case 37 Splenic Trauma

Figure 37.4

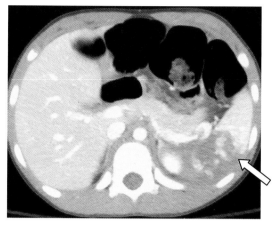

Figure 37.5

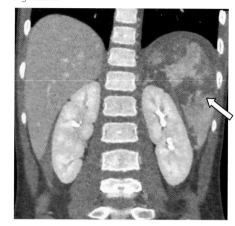

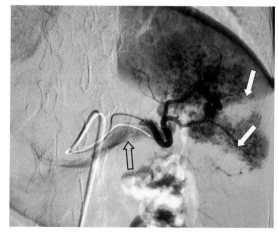

Figure 37.6

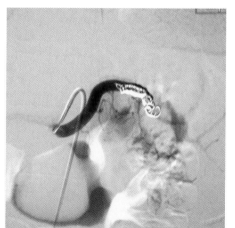

Figure 37.7

Findings

▶ Axial and coronal enhanced computed tomography (CT) images (Figs. 37.4 and 37.5) demonstrate a splenic laceration with involvement of the hilar vessels.

▶ Splenic angiogram (Fig. 37.6) shows early draining splenic vein (hollow arrow), consistent with traumatic arteriovenous fistula. Note the heterogenous perfusion of the spleen with areas of poorly perfused parenchyma (arrows).

▶ Coil embolization of the splenic artery distal to the origin of the dorsal pancreatic was performed to stasis (Fig. 37.7).

Teaching Points

▶ The spleen is the most frequently injured intraperitoneal organ following blunt abdominal trauma.

▶ Categories of splenic injury from the American Academy of Surgery and Trauma Organ Injury scale:

    I—subcapsular hematoma <25% surface area, capsular tear <1 cm of parenchymal depth

    II—subcapsular hematoma 25%–50% of surface area, intraparenchymal hematoma < 5cm in diameter; 1–3 cm laceration without involvement of trabecular vessels

    III—subcapsular hematoma >50% of surface area, intraparenchymal hematoma >10 cm; laceration >3 cm parenchymal depth with involvement of trabecular vessels

IV—laceration involving segmental/hilar vessels with >25% devascularization

V—completely shattered spleen, total splenic devascularization

► When no active extravasation is identified, proximal embolization to decrease perfusion pressure of the spleen is performed to stop hemorrhage. Collateral blood flow to the splenic parenchyma from short gastric and capsular arteries usually prevents total splenic infarction. In the setting of discrete extravasation, subselective embolization may be performed.

► When possible, embolization of the splenic artery embolization should be distal to the dorsal pancreatic artery, which typically arises from the proximal third of the splenic artery.

Treatment

► Patients who remain hemodynamically unstable after resuscitation should be managed surgically.

► The indications for splenic artery embolization vary but include ongoing hemorrhage in a hemodynamically stable patient, and imaging findings of contrast extravasation or direct vascular injury, with a high grade of injury.

Further Reading

Imbrogno BF, Ray CE. Splenic artery embolization in blunt trauma. *Semin Intervent Radiol.* 2012; 29(2):147–149.

History

▶ Fevers and Leukocytosis 1 Week after Gastrectomy Complicated by Abscess

After removal of the drainage catheter, the patient became hypotensive and tachycardic, and a computed tomography (CT) (Fig. 38.3) was obtained.

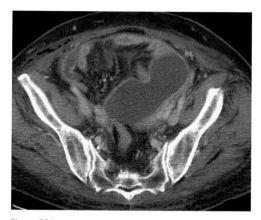

Figure 38.1

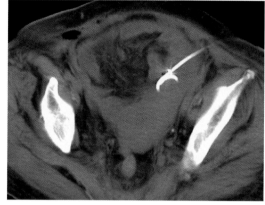

Figure 38.2

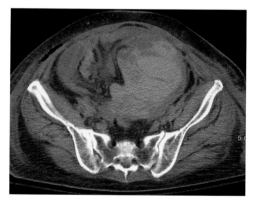

Figure 38.3

Case 38 Drainage of Abdominal Abscess Complicated by Inferior Epigastric Artery Injury Pseudoaneurysm

Figure 38.4

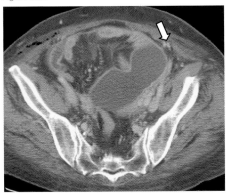

Figure 38.5

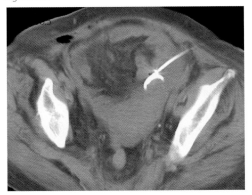

Figure 38.6

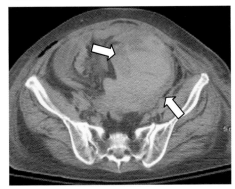

Figure 38.7

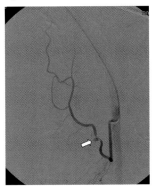

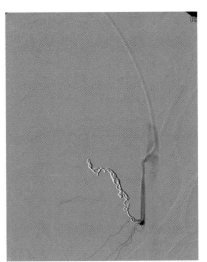

Figure 38.8

Findings

▶ A bilobed collection with an enhancing rim is seen in the left lower quadrant Fig. 38.4. Percutaneous drainage was performed (Fig. 38.5), inadvertently crossing the inferior epigastric vessels (arrow, Fig. 38.4).

▶ CT performed immediately after catheter removal (Fig. 38.6) when the patient became hypotensive shows hyperdense intraabdominal hematoma at the site of the previous collection (arrows).

▶ Left inferior epigastric angiogram (Fig. 38.7) shows a focal pseudoaneurysm where the catheter had crossed the vessel (arrow). This was successfully embolized with 3–5 mm stainless steel coils (Fig. 37.8).

Teaching Points

▶ Preprocedure planning must include a careful review of available imaging and consideration of interpositioned normal anatomic structures to minimize the risk of injury or complication.

▶ The inferior epigastric artery is a distal branch of the external iliac artery. Because of the proximity to the common femoral artery which is typically accessed for lower-extremity intervention, catheterization of the inferior epigastric artery is best performed from a contralateral approach.

▶ A pseudoaneurysm is an injury to at least one layer of the arterial wall. Whereas a true aneurysm may be treated by occluding the sac, there is no "sac" in a pseudoaneurysm because it represents a contained rupture.

▶ Most reported cases of inferior epigastric pseudoaneuryms are iatrogenic, related to abdominal wall procedures including hernia repair, surgical drains, and trocar injury during laparoscopy.

Management

▶ Embolization of a pseudoaneurysm should include the vessel immediately distal and proximal to the injury to prevent revascularization from collateral vessels.

▶ Alternative treatment options include ultrasound-guided thrombin injection in larger lesions, or surgical ligation.

Further Reading

Georgiadis GS, Souftas VD, Papas TT, et al. Inferior epigastric artery false aneurysms: review of the literature and case report. *Eur J Vasc Endovasc Surg.* 2007; 33(2):182–186.

History

▸ A 45-Year-Old Female with History of Roux-en-Y Gastric Bypass Presents with Melena

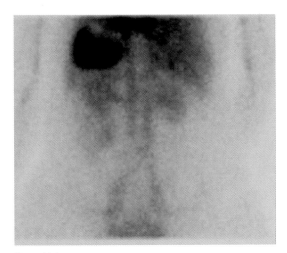

Figure 39.1

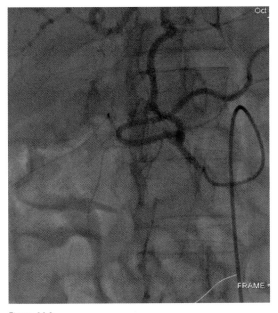

Figure 39.2

Case 39   Upper Gastrointestinal Bleed

Figure 39.3

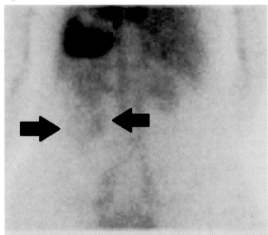

Figure 39.4

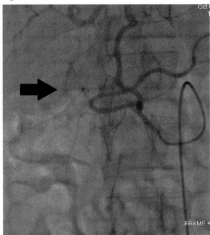

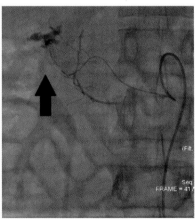

Figure 39.5

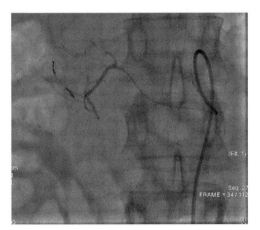

Figure 39.6

Findings

▸ Figure 39.3 represents a tagged red blood cell scan showing radiotracer activity in the right upper quadrant (black arrow). Cine images (not shown) demonstrate increased pooling and movement of the activity across to the left abdomen.

▸ Selective angiogram of the inferior pancreaticoduodenal artery arising from the superior mesenteric artery (Fig. 39.4) shows active contrast extravasation (black arrow).

▸ Superselective arteriogram of a branch of the pancreaticoduodenal artery shows contrast extravasation into the duodenum (black arrow in Fig. 39.5).

▸ Figure 39.6 shows successful coil embolization and exclusion of the bleeding branch.

Teaching Points

▸ Common causes of acute upper gastrointestinal bleeding include peptic ulcer disease, variceal bleeding, gastritis, Mallory Weiss tears, postoperative marginal ulcers, and iatrogenic causes such as after an endoscopic sphincterotomy.

- Radionuclide scintigraphy is most commonly performed with ^{99}Tc-labeled red blood cells with the ability to detect bleeding as slow as 0.4 mL/min. ^{99}Tc-labeled red blood cell scans are more sensitive than catheter angiography, which detects bleeding at a rate of 0.1 to 1.0 mL/min. Additionally, the chance of identifying hemorrhage on a ^{99}Tc-labeled red blood cell scan is higher because it can be imaged over several hours compared to angiography, which images over a few seconds.

Management

- Endoscopic diagnosis and management with clipping or cauterization is effective in the majority of cases of upper gastrointestinal bleeding. Cases refractory to endoscopic techniques or unreachable by endoscopic techniques can be treated with angiography and embolization. In this case, secondary to the Roux-en-Y anatomy, the endoscopist could not reach the bleeding segment.
- In cases with a negative angiogram, empiric embolization of the gastroduodenal artery or left gastric artery (depending on cause and findings on endoscopy) is often successful in treatment of the acute episode and prevents recurrent bleeding.
- Embolization can be performed with microcoils, gelfoam, polyvinyl alcohol particles, or glue.

Further Reading

Loffror R, Rao P, Ota S, et al. Embolization of acute nonvariceal upper gastrointestinal hemorrhage resistant to endoscopic treatment: results and predictors of recurrent bleeding. *Cardiovasc Intervent Radiol.* 2010; 33:1088–1100.

History

▶ A 60-Year-Old Male with Acute Lower Gastrointestinal Bleeding (Radionuclide Scanning Was Unavailable)

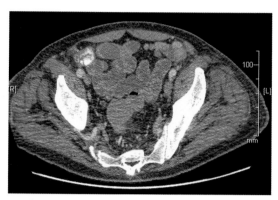

Figure 40.1

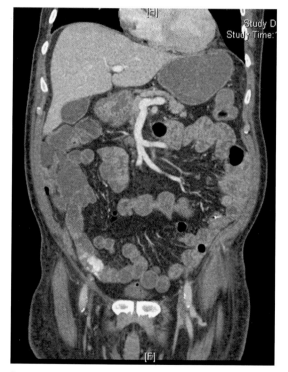

Figure 40.2

Case 40 Lower Gastrointestinal Bleed

Figure 40.3

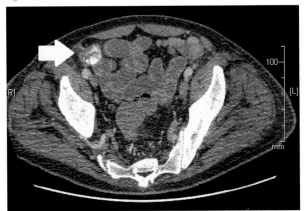

Figure 40.4

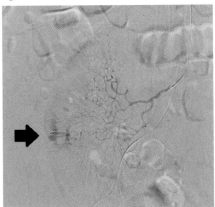

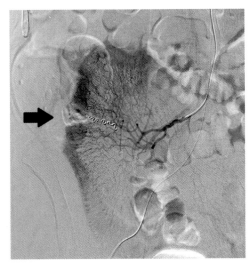

Figure 40.5

Findings

▶ Figures 40.2 and 40.3 demonstrate intraluminal contrast in the right colon representing active bleeding (white arrow).

▶ Superior mesenteric angiogram (Fig. 40.4) demonstrates active bleeding originating from a branch of the right colic artery corresponding to the finding on computed tomography (CT) (black arrow).

▶ Postembolization angiogram (Fig. 40.5) shows successful coil embolization (black arrow) of the distal offending arterial branch.

Teaching Points

▶ Common causes of lower gastrointestinal bleeding include diverticulosis, angiodysplasia, and cancer/polyps.

▶ When patients are stable and the site of bleeding is in question, radionuclide scintigraphy (^{99}Tc-labeled red blood cell scan) or CT angiography may be helpful. Lower gastrointestinal bleeding is intermittent and often self-limited, and tagged red cell scans that are more sensitive than angiography at detecting hemorrhage can be very useful.

- CT angiography can identify potential cause of lower gastrointestinal bleeding with ~90% accuracy.
- When patients are hypotensive and have transfusion requirements of more than 5 units, the likelihood of a positive angiogram is high and immediate angiography or colonoscopy (without tagged red cell scan or CT) should be performed.
- The use of provocative angiography, injection of a thrombolytic agent, heparin, or vasodilators into the target vessel of suspicion to identify lesions not seen with standard angiography is controversial.

Management

- Transarterial embolization with microcoils, gelfoam, or polyvinyl alcohol particles is very effective in controlling acute bleeding.
- Selective embolization at the level of the vasa recta should be performed to decrease the risk of bowel ischemia.
- While embolization can be effective in controlling acute bleeding, the risk of recurrent bleeding in the setting of angiodysplasia or arteriovenous malformations is high, and resection should be considered.

Further Reading

Marti M, Artigas JM, Garzon G, et al. Acute lower intestinal bleeding: feasibility and diagnostic performance of CT angiography. *Radiology*. 2012; 262:109–116.
Strate LL, Naumann CR. The role of colonoscopy and radiological procedures in the management of acute lower intestinal bleeding. *Clin Gastroenterol Hepatol.* 2010; 8:333–343.

History

▶ A 13-Year-Old Boy with Recurrent Nosebleeds

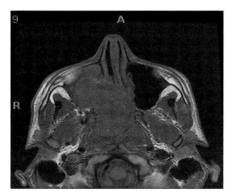

Figure 41.1

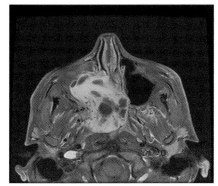

Figure 41.2

Case 41   Juvenile Nasal Angiofibroma

Figure 41.3

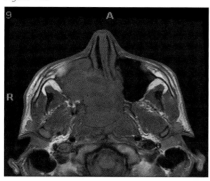

Figure 41.4

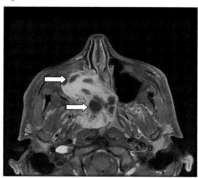

Figure 41.5

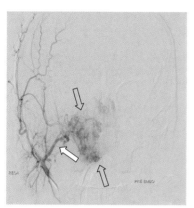

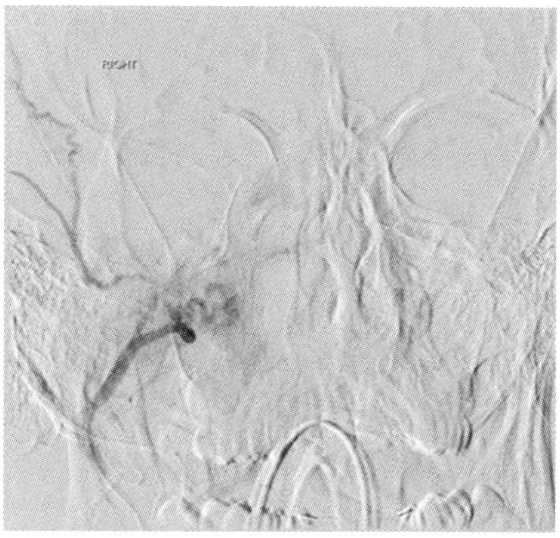

Figure 41.6

Findings

▶ Precontrast T1-weighted magnetic resonance (MR) (Fig. 41.3) demonstrates a heterogenous right-sided nasopharyngeal mass that exerts mass effect on the nasopharyngeal space and is associated with bone erosion of the sphenoid sinus.

▶ The mass enhances intensely with contrast (Fig. 41.4). Note the large flow voids within the mass (arrows).

▶ Right external carotid arteriography (Fig. 41.5) shows the hypervascular mass (hollow arrows) arising from the maxillary artery (arrow).

▶ After distal embolization with polyvinyl alcohol particles (Fig. 41.6), there is stasis within the branches of the maxillary artery previously seen to supply the tumor.

Teaching Points

▶ Juvenile nasal angiofibroma occurs in the second decade almost exclusively in males and is the most common benign nasopharyngeal tumor.

▶ While histologically benign, these tumors are locally destructive and have a tendency to erode bone, typically into the sinuses or orbit.

▶ Patients commonly present with recurrent epistaxis, which may be severe, and/or signs of nasal obstruction.

Management

▶ Preoperative embolization may be performed to decrease intraoperative blood loss. Tumors are typically supplied by branches of the ipsilateral external carotid artery, but large tumors may also derive supply from the ipsilateral internal carotid artery and also occasionally by branches of the contralateral carotid arteries.

- Ideally, surgery should occur within 3 days following the procedure to prevent revascularization of the tumor by collateral vessels.
- Prior to embolization of a target artery, careful study is imperative to ensure there are no ophthalmic artery branches to avoid nontarget embolization that could result in vision loss.

Further Reading

Wu AW, Mowry SE, Vinuela F, et al. Bilateral vascular supply in juvenile nasopharyngeal angiofibromas. *Laryngoscope*. 2011; 121(3):639–643.

History

▶ A 12-Year-Old Boy with Painful, Swollen Left Testicle

What is the diagnosis and what are the treatment options?

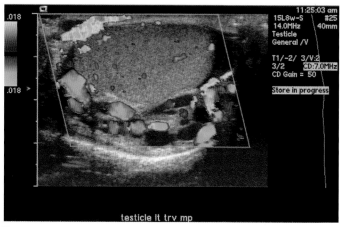

Figure 42.1

Case 42 Male Varicocele Embolized with Coils and Sclerosant

Figure 42.2

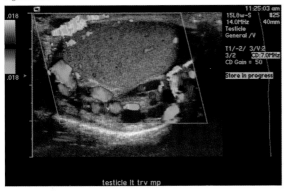

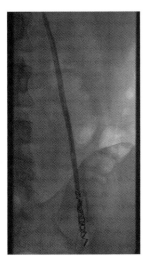

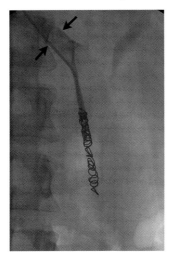

Figure 42.3

Figure 42.4

Findings

▶ Ultrasound demonstrates dilatation of venous sinuses of the pampiniform plexus (Fig. 42.2, arrows).

▶ The left internal spermatic vein (ISV) has been catheterized from the left renal vein (Fig. 42.3). Distal coils are seen at the level of the sacroiliac joint. After the distal coils were placed, sodium tetradecyl sulfate was injected, and a second level of coils was placed approximately 2 cm from the confluence of the internal spermatic vein with the left renal vein (Fig. 42.4), which is marked by arrows.

Teaching Points

▶ Doppler ultrasound is the modality of choice for diagnosing varicoceles. In addition to dilation of the pampiniform plexus, findings include continuous reflux and high peak retrograde flow in the ISV.

▶ The majority (>80%) of primary varicoceles are either left sided or bilateral, due to the relatively high impedence of the left renal vein compared to the inferior vena cava (into which the right internal spermatic vein drains).

▶ For this reason, unilateral right-sided varicoceles are uncommon and warrant further evaluation for mechanical obstruction by retroperitoneal or abdominal tumors (i.e. secondary varicocele).

- In standard anatomy, the right ISV drains directly into the inferior vena cava just below the renal vein, and the left drains into the left renal vein. Variations are common; they are seen in approximately 20% of patients.
- Indications for treatment of varicoceles include pain, infertility, and/or testicular atrophy.

Management

- Valsalva maneuver or reverse Trendelenberg position may help document incompetent valves during venography.
- Treatment options include surgery (open, laparoscopic, or microsurgery) or transcatheter embolization. Both are generally performed as outpatient procedures, with comparable success and rates of recurrence. Recurrence after surgery may be treated with transcatheter embolization and vice versa.
- Transcatheter embolization can be performed utilizing a combination of coils and/or a sclerosant such as sodium tetradecyl sulfate made into a foam by mixture with sterile saline or Ethiodol and air.
- When a sclerosant is used, care must be taken to prevent reflux into the left renal vein. The most distal coils are placed just above inguinal ligament or pubic symphysis and the most proximal in the ISV 1–2 cm from the confluence with the renal vein to prevent recanalization from parallel, capsular, and colic collaterals. Additional coils may be placed in between to prevent recanalization from pelvic collaterals.
- Some patients may experience temporary scrotal swelling and pain after embolization. Treatment includes oral nonsteroidal antiinflammatory drugs.
- Because the treatment is usually performed on children or men being treated for infertility, minimizing radiation exposure is important. Use of "last-image hold" or "fluoro-store" images rather than photospot imaging can decrease exposure up to 25-fold.

Further Reading

Iaccarino V, Venetucci P. Interventional radiology of mal varicocele: current status. *Cardiovasc Intervent Radiol*. 2012; 35(6):1263–1280.

Masson P, Brannigan RE. The varicocele. *Urol Clin North Am*. 2014; 41(1):129–144.

History

▶ A 30 year-old male patient with known history of paroxysmal nocturnal haemoglobinuria (PNH) and symptomatic cholelithiasis was scheduled for an elective laparoscopic cholecystectomy. Why is this procedure being performed?

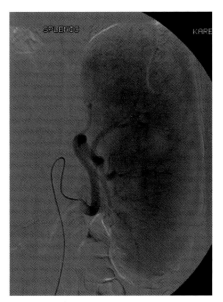

Figure 43.1

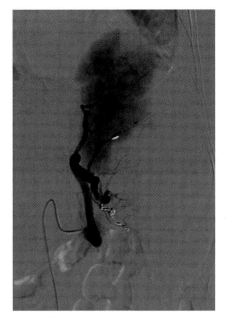

Figure 43.2

Case 43   Partial Splenic Embolization

Figure 43.3

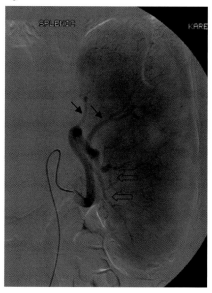

Figure 43.4

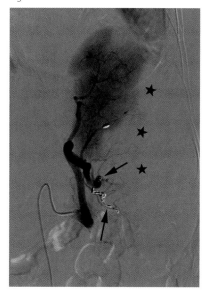

Figure 43.5

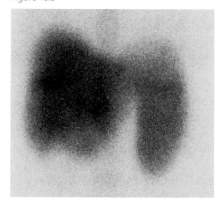

Figure 43.6

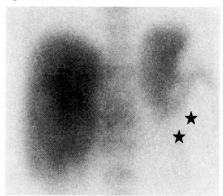

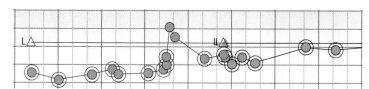

Figure 43.7

Findings

▶ Preembolization digital subtraction selective splenic arteriogram shows an enlarged spleen with normal vascularity (Fig. 43.3). The splenic artery divides into superior (black arrows) and inferior (hollow arrows) terminal branches near splenic hilum.

▶ Digital subtraction splenic arteriogram obtained after embolization of approximately 70% of spleen (Fig. 43.4) shows embolization coils in the inferior splenic artery branches (arrows). Lack of parenchymal blush (stars) is now seen in inferior portion of the spleen.

▶ Tc99m sulfur colloid nuclear scan before (Fig. 43.5) and after (Fig. 43.6) partial splenic embolization shows lack of parenchymal uptake in the lower aspect of the spleen (stars) due to partial splenic infarction.

▶ Platelet count trend before and after embolization showing improvement in the platelet count after partial splenic artery embolization (Fig. 43.7), allowing laparoscopic cholecystectomy to be performed with a lower risk of bleeding. There is often a rebound elevation of platelet count that peaks at 2–4 weeks following embolization.

Teaching Points

▶ Paroxysmal nocturnal hemoglobinuria (PNH) is a rare acquired nonmalignant stem cell disorder, that occurs mainly in young adults and is characterized by intravascular hemolysis, hemoglobinuria cytopenias, and despite thrombocytopenia there is an an increased risk of life-threatening thrombotic events.

▶ Thrombocytopenia was thought to be secondary to hypersplenism. Partial splenic artery embolization was performed to optimize the platelet count prior to elective surgery.

▶ Prior to coil placement, embolization was performed with particles for terminal vessel blockade. Embolization of the more proximal splenic arteries with coils alone would not cause infarction of splenic tissue due to the presence of collateral vessels, principally via the short gastric and capsular arteries.

▶ Partial splenic embolization reduces sequestration and destruction of the blood elements, while maintaining the opsonization function of the spleen.

Management

▶ Embolization of 50%–70% of splenic volume is performed, preferably of the lower pole both to minimize diaphragmatic irritation resulting in pain and associated sympathetic pleural effusion/atelectasis and to allow for easier drainage of abscess should one develop.

▶ Complication of splenic embolization includes abscess formation, splenic rupture, necrosis of the gastric wall, renal insufficiency, acute pancreatitis, splenic vein thrombosis, postembolization pain, sepsis, and pneumonia.

▶ Postembolization abdominal pain is usually well controlled by medication. Continuous epidural analgesia has been also used.

▶ The local effect of arterial embolization on the spleen can be assessed by nuclear medicine studies (Technetium-99 sulfur colloid scan), computed tomography (CT), ultrasound, or magnetic resonance imaging (MRI); however, clinical success is judged by improvement in platelet count.

Further Reading

Krishnan SK, Hill A, Hillmen P, et al. Improving cytopenia with splenic artery embolization in a patient with paroxysmal nocturnal hemoglobinuria on eculizumab. *Int J Hematol*. 2013; 98(6):716–8. doi: 10.1007/s12185-013-1454-1.

Madoff DC, Denys A, Wallace MJ, et al. Splenic arterial interventions: anatomy, indications, technical considerations, and potential complications. *Radiographics*. 2005; 25:S191–S211.

Rotoli B, Luzzatto L. Paroxysmal nocturnal hemoglobinuria. *Baillieres Clin Haematol*. 1989; 2:113–138.

History

▶ After embolization of the gastroduodenal artery for active extravasation (not shown), an angiogram is done. What happened and what are the treatment options?

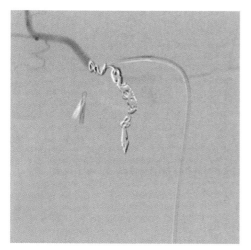

Figure 44.1

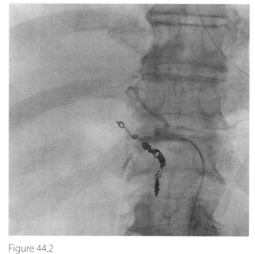

Figure 44.2

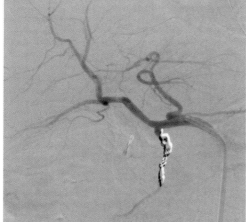

Figure 44.3

Case 44 Retrieval of Nontarget Coil

Figure 44.4

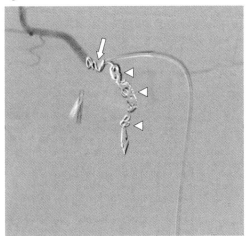

Figure 44.5

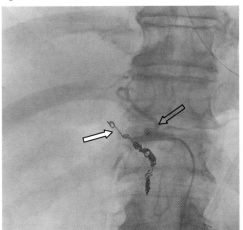

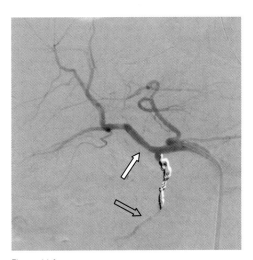

Figure 44.6

Findings

▶ Hepatic angiogram and after coil embolization of a gastroduodenal artery, pseudoaneurysm (not shown) demonstrates a coil that has migrated into the right hepatic artery (Fig. 44.4, arrow). Based on the position of the catheter and the right hepatic artery, the expected course of the gastroduodenal artery (now packed with coils) is shown by the arrowheads.

▶ Unsubtracted digital angiogram with the catheter in the common hepatic artery (Fig. 44.5) shows early takeoff of the left hepatic artery proximal to the gastroduodenal artery (hollow arrow). Note again the malpositioned coil in the course of the right hepatic artery (arrow).

▶ The migrated coil was snared (not shown) and removed, after which there is restoration of antegrade flow in the right hepatic artery (arrow, Fig. 44.6). Distal to the nest of coils, the gastroduodenal artery is reconstitued (hollow arrow) by the inferior pancreaticoduodenal arteries arising from the superior mesenteric artery.

Teaching Points

▶ Coil migration can occur when the diameter of the coil is either too small or too large to form in the target vessel, or if the coil is too long. A rule of thumb is to choose a coil that is 10% larger than the diameter of the target vessel.

▶ In situations where coil migration can have potentially catastrophic consequences, use of detachable coils should be considered. For example, when occluding the feeding artery of a pulmonary arteriovenous malformation, if a coil were to pass through the malformation, it would pass into the left heart via the pulmonary vein and cause paradoxical embolism such as a cerebrovascular event.

Management

▶ Coils come in a variety of diameters, lengths, and shapes, both with and without dacron fibrils. It is important to remember that the coils themselves do not occlude the vessel, but the slow flow they create and the fibrils promote thrombosis, which can take a few minutes to occur. Tincture of time rather than placing coils one after another ultimately saves time, reduces cost, and minimizes the risk of coil migration.

▶ When not contraindicated, anticoagulation should be considered at the time a coil is placed in a nontarget vessel to prevent non-target vessel occlusion while retrieval is attempted.

▶ Devices used for retrieval include snares (multiloop snares are particularly useful for intravascular retrieval) and alligator forceps.

▶ In this case, if the coil had not been successfully retrieved, inadvertant embolization of the right hepatic artery in the setting of a patent portal vein is unlikely to have been clinically significant.

Further Reading

Egglin TK, Dickey KW, Rosenblatt M, et al. Retrieval of intravascular foreign bodies: experience in 32 cases. *Am J Roentgenol.* 1995; 164(5):1259–1264.

History

▶ A 70-Year-Old Female with Pelvic Mass Presents with Anuria and Increasing Creatinine

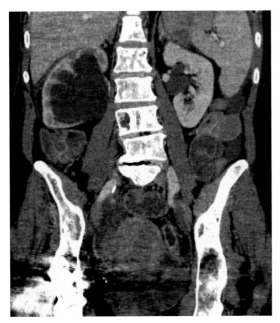

Figure 45.1

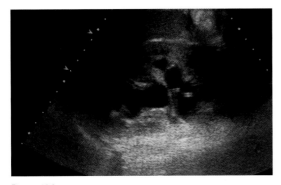

Figure 45.2

Case 45   Hydronephrosis from Obstructing Mass Failing Ureteral Stent

Figure 45.3

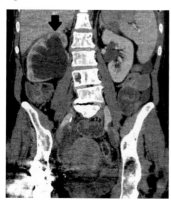

Figure 45.4

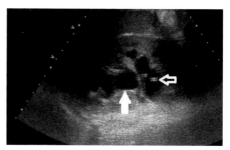

Figure 45.5

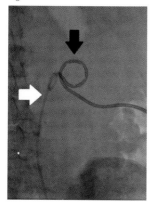

Figure 45.6

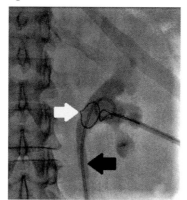

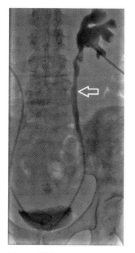

Figure 45.7

Findings

▶ Coronal computed tomography (CT) scan (Fig. 45.3) demonstrates marked hydronephrosis of the right kidney (arrows) with obstructing pelvic mass. Ureteral stents were placed cystocopically; however, creatinine remained elevated with persistent hydronephrosis (white arrow) on follow-up ultrasound (Fig. 45.4). Note the ureteral stent on ultrasound (open arrow).

▶ A nephrostomy tube was placed (Fig. 45.5, black arrow) and the proximal portion of the ureteral stent is seen (white arrow).

▶ Figure 45.6 demonstrates intraprocedural snare retrieval of the cystoscopically placed ureteral stent (black arrow). A snare is looped around the proximal pigtail of the ureteral stent (white arrow).

▶ Figure 45.7 demonstrates a nephroureterostomy tube in place (open arrow) with pigtails formed in the renal pelvis and bladder.

Teaching Points

▶ In patients with normal bladders who require urinary drainage, cystoscopic ureteral stent placement should be attempted first for patient comfort and safety.

▶ In the event of sepsis or failed ureteral stent placement, nephrostomy or nephroureterostomy catheters can be placed. Nephroureterostomy catheters are preferred in most situations because they can be capped to allow for internal drainage and the length of catheter minimizes the risk of inadvertent dislodgement.

▶ In certain situations, however, nephrostomy is favored over nephroureterostomy. These include (1) urinary diversion to prevent urine from entering the bladder (e.g., in the presence of a vesicovaginal fistula), (2) to relieve debilitating bladder spasm associated with nephroureterostomy or stent, and (3) bladder hemorrhage that is exacerbated by the presence of a catheter.

▶ Ureteral stents can be removed cystoscopically or through the nephrostomy tract. In this case, the advantage to the latter is twofold: (1) access across the obstruction is maintained, facilitating nephroureterostomy catheter placement; and (2) it is done by a single operator in a single procedure.

▶ Ureteral stents should not be placed in patients who are unable to void spontaneously or who are incontinent.

▶ Ureteral stents should also not be placed in patients who have neo-bladders or conduits because the mucus secreted by the bowel quickly occludes the distal holes in the catheter.

Management

▶ Nephrostomy, nephroureterostomy, and ureteral tubes/stents should be exchanged every 3–6 months to prevent occlusion.

▶ The use of prophylactic antibiotics for routine exchange is controversial.

Further Reading

Dyer RB, Regan JD, Kavanagh PV, et al. Percutaneous nephrostomy with extensions of the technique: step by step. *Radiographics*. 2002; *22*:503–525.

History

▶ Cervical Cancer. Pulsatile Blood Seen during Retrograde Exchange of Indwelling Ureteral Stent

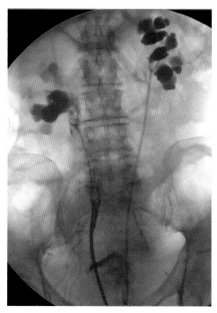

Figure 46.1

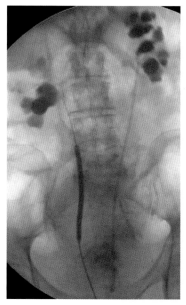

Figure 46.2

Case 46   Ureteral-Right Iliac Artery Fistula

Figure 46.3

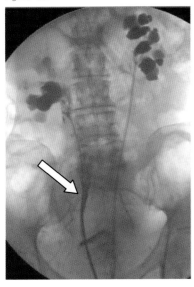

Figure 46.4

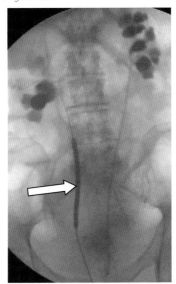

Figure 46.5

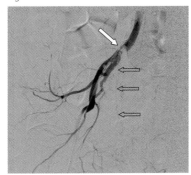

Figure 46.6

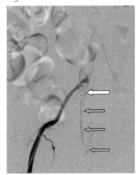

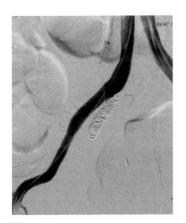

Figure 46.7

Findings

► Retrograde injection of contrast into the right ureter at the time of stent exchange demonstrates filling of branches of the right iliac artery (Fig. 46.3, arrow).

► A balloon has been placed over a wire and inflated (Fig. 46.4, arrow) to tamponade and prevent further extravasation after the stent was removed.

► Digital subtraction angiography of the right iliac artery shows a filling defect (Fig. 46.5, arrow) consistent with clot at the bifurcation into the internal and external iliac arteries. Though largely subtracted, the course of the balloon in the ureter can be seen crossing the artery at exactly this level (hollow arrows).

► After thrombectomy and coil embolization of the internal iliac artery (Fig. 46.6, arrow) to prevent retrograde endoleak, right iliac angiogram shows extravasation into the ureter (hollow arrows).

► A covered stent was placed (Fig. 46.7) extending from the common iliac to the external iliac artery, spanning the fistula; there is no further extravasation seen.

Teaching Points

► Uretero-arterial fistulae are most commonly seen in patients who have undergone either abdominal/pelvic surgery or radiation therapy and have chronic ureteral stents.

► The common iliac artery bifurcation is the most common site of fistula formation because it is where the ureter crosses immediately anterior to the artery.

► Uretero-arterial fistulae are notoriously difficult to diagnose and should be suspected in patients at high risk who have persistent hematuria and no other identifiable source.

Management

► Morbidity related to uretero-arterial fistula is high; once identified, it should be treated urgently with either placement of a stent graft across the fistula, as in this case, or open surgical repair.

► Surgical repair is often difficult because most patients have adhesions from having undergone previous surgery and/or radiation. Surgical repair, either uretero-ureterostomy or nephrectomy, is usually reserved for failure or recurrence after endovascular treatment.

► Prophylactic antibiotics should be considered because of the communication between potentially colonized urine and the bloodstream.

Further Reading

Tselikas L, Pellerin O, Di Primio M, et al. Uretero-iliac fistula: modern treatment via the endovascular route. *Diagn Interv Imaging*. 2013; 94(3):311–318.

History

▶ Bladder Cancer Status post Cystectomy and Ileal Conduit Complicated by Bilateral Uretero-Enteric Anastomotic Strictures. What catheters are shown in Figure 47.3?

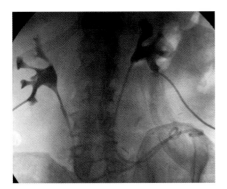

Figure 47.1

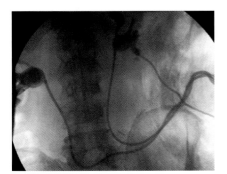

Figure 47.2

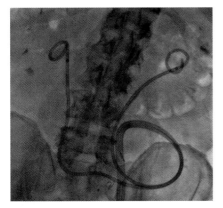

Figure 47.3

Case 47 Retrograde Nephrostomy Catheters

Figure 47.4

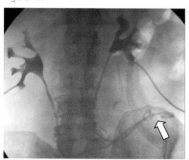

Figure 47.5

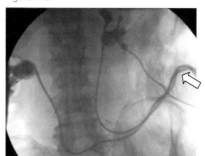

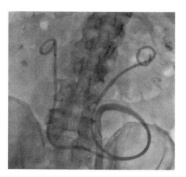

Figure 47.6

Findings

▸ Bilateral nephroureteral catheters have been placed with the distal pigtails in the ileal conduit (Fig. 47.4, arrow).

▸ Each catheter has been advanced through the conduit and out of the stoma located in the left lower quadrant (Fig. 47.5, arrow).

▸ Both catheters have been converted to retrograde nephrostomy catheters with the retention pigtails in the renal pelvis. The catheters now drain into the stoma. The antegrade nephrostomy catheters have been removed.

Teaching Points

▸ Retrograde catheters are ideal for patients with ureteral obstruction after cystectomy and ileal conduit because they drain into the stoma bag instead of antegrade nephrostomy catheters that require an additional bags for drainage.

▸ Nephroureteral catheters in nonnative bladders (e.g., ileal conduits, neobladder, etc.) that are created from bowel can neither be capped nor stented because the bowel secretes mucus that occludes the sideholes of the catheter.

Management

▸ After obtaining "through-and-through" access from the site of antegrade access out of the stoma with an angiographic catheter, a stiff wire is advanced from the stoma side out of the antegrade nephrostomy tract. A retrograde nephrostomy can be placed over the wire and formed in the renal pelvis as the wire is pulled back.

- Routine exchange of all urinary drainage catheters (nephrostomy, nephroureteral catheter, ureteral stent, retrograde nephrostomy) is necessary to minimize the risk of catheter occlusion and resulting urosepsis. Typical routine exchange intervals range from 3 to 6 months.
- For patients who tend to have encrusted catheters, a sidehole may be made in the shaft of the catheter prior to placement. This functions as an "escape route" for the next exchange, allowing for a wire to be advanced out of the catheter and up into the renal pelvis to preserve access if a wire cannot be advanced out of the end of the catheter due to encrustation.
- The need for antibiotic prophylaxis prior to routine exchange is controvertial but widely practiced.

Further Reading

Adamo R, Saad WE, Brown DB. Management of nephrostomy drains and ureteral stents. *Tech Vasc Interv Radiol.* 2009;12(3):193–204.

Alago W Jr, Sofocleous CT, Covey AM, et al. Placement of transileal conduit retrograde nephroureteral stents in patients with ureteral obstruction after cystectomy: technique and outcome. *Am J Roentgenol.* 2008; 191(5):1536–1539.

History

▶ A 68-Year-Old Female with Ovarian Cancer and Ureteral Obstruction

Both tubes have been capped for 2 weeks and she has not had pain, fever, or elevation in serum creatinine. What is the best option for eliminating the external tubes?

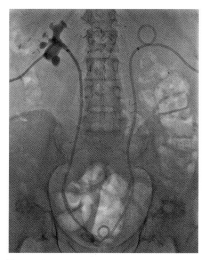

Figure 48.1

Case 48 Ureteral Stent

Figure 48.2

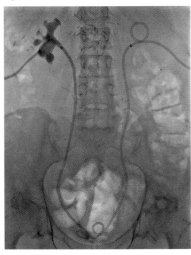

Figure 48.3

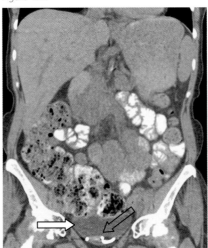

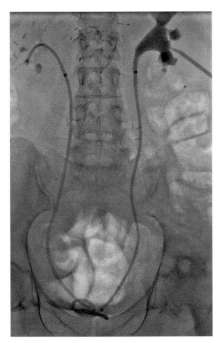

Figure 48.4

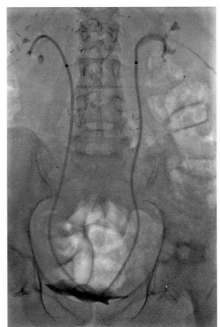

Figure 48.5

Findings

▶ Contrast injection into the left nephroureteral catheter shows minimal hydronephrosis (Fig. 48.2). The proximal pigtail is formed in the renal pelvis and the distal pigtail in the bladder. A right-sided nephroureteral catheter is also seen.

▶ Coronal computed tomography (CT) reformat (Fig. 48.3) shows the distal pigtails of the nephroureteral catheters (hollow arrow) in the normal-appearing bladder (arrow).

▶ Both nephroureteral catheters have been exchanged over wire for double J stents. Contrast injection into a catheter in the right renal pelvis (Fig. 48.4) confirms there is good drainage across the stent into the bladder.

Five minutes later, another image was obtained (Fig. 48.5) showing the contrast has drained across the stent into the bladder.

Teaching Points

▶ In patients who have normal bladders, cystoscopic stent placement is favored because drainage can be achieved through a normal orifice without the need for transparenchymal access.

▶ Patients with urinary obstruction who fail or are not candidates for cystoscopic stent placement may be treated with percutaneous nephrostomy or nephroureterostomy placement. If a patients tolerates capping trial of a nephroureterostomy, as in this case, stent placement should be considered.

▶ Over-the-wire exchange of a nephroureteral catheter for a stent is performed by "pushing" the stent into position. This can be done with the prepackaged device or by using a standard nephrostomy tube. The latter is preferred if ongoing external access is needed (e.g., if there is blood in the system after stent placement, the antegrade nephrostomy catheter can allow drainage until it resolves).

▶ If a primary stent is placed (i.e., stent placement at the time of first antegrade access), a "covering" nephrostomy may be left in place until function of the ureteral stent is confirmed. Because the pigtails of the nephrostomy and stent can intertwine, removal of the nephrostomy over a wire and under fluoroscopic visualization is advisable.

▶ Primary stents should *not* be placed if there is significant clot in the collecting system related to antegrade access. Conversion could be attempted after a short period, usually 1–2 weeks, after hematuria has cleared.

Management

▶ Ureteral stents are generally exchanged every 3–6 months to prevent encrustation or infection. In women this can be done either fluoroscopically or at cystoscopy. In men, the length of the penile urethra increases the likelihood of losing access fluoroscopically, and therefore cystoscopic exchange is preferred.

▶ Stents are available with different sidehole configurations. In the setting of a ureteral leak, a stent or catheter with sideholes only in the proximal or distal pigtail (i.e., not along the ureteral portion) will help divert urine from the site of leakage.

Further Reading

Hausegger KA, Portugaller HR. Percutaneous nephrostomy and antegrade ureteral stenting: technique-indications-complications. *Eur Radiol.* 2006; 16(9):2016–2030.

History

▶ Failed Cystoscopic Exchange of Occluded Ureteral Stent. What is the Best Alternative Option for Urinary Drainage?

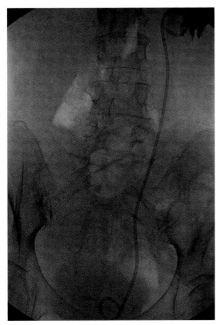

Figure 49.1

Case 49 Routine Transurethral Exchange of Ureteral Stent

Figure 49.2

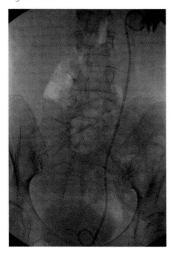

Figure 49.3

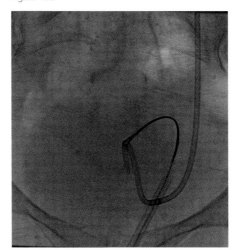

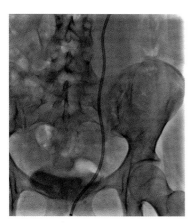

Figure 49.4

Findings

▶ Indwelling ureteral stent is positioned with pigtails in the renal pelvis and bladder (Fig. 49.2).

▶ In Figure 49.3, a snare has been advanced through a sheath placed into the bladder via the urethra. The snare has been used to capture the distal pigtail of the ureteral stent (Fig. 49.3). The stent is then pulled out through the sheath (Fig. 49.4) and exchanged over a wire for new.

Teaching Points

▶ Stents are only indicated in the setting of a native bladder. Neobladders and conduits created from small bowel secrete mucus, which quickly occludes the distal sideholes in stents placed in these nonnative bladders.

▶ Depending on the size of the cystoscope, larger stents may be difficult for urologists to exchange at cystoscopy.

▶ When using this technique of transurethral snare and exchange in men, care must be taken not to lose access to the ureter when pulling the catheter through the penile urethra.

Management

▶ Ureteral stents require routine exchange every 3–6 months. This may be performed cystoscopically by urologists or fluoroscopically by interventional radiologists.

▶ Results of self-expanding metallic stents placed for malignant ureteral obstruction have been disappointing with early occlusion due to urothelial hyperplasia and encrustation.

▶ Tumor, chemotherapy, and radiation therapy all contribute to periureteric fibrosis. Once a stent is placed in this setting, stent removal is unusual.

▶ In some tumors, for example, lymphoma, fibrosis may not occur and once the obstructing lesion has resolved a trial of stent removal may be considered.

Further Reading

Park SW, Cha IH, Hong SJ, et al. Fluoroscopy-guided transurethral removal and exchange of ureteral stents in female patients: technical notes. *J Vasc Interv Radiol.* 2007; 18(2):251–256.

- In certain situations, however, nephrostomy is favored over nephroureterostomy. These include (1) urinary diversion to prevent urine from entering the bladder (e.g., in the presence of a vesicovaginal fistula), (2) to relieve debilitating bladder spasm associated with nephroureterostomy or stent, and (3) bladder hemorrhage that is exacerbated by the presence of a catheter.
- Ureteral stents may be removed from the bladder by cystoscopy, or from the renal pelvis, as in this case. In this case, the advantage to the latter is twofold: (1) access across the obstruction is maintained, facilitating nephroureterostomy catheter placement; and (2) it is done by a single operator in a single procedure.

Management

- Routine exchange of urinary drainage catheters is required every 3–6 months to prevent catheter occlusion.
- Unlike most drainage catheters, in abscesses or the biliary tree for example, urinary drainage catheters do not require routine forward flushes.
- Nephroureterostomy catheters may be capped, rendering their function that of a ureteral stent. If a patient tolerates this without pain, fever, or pericatheter leakage, conversion to a ureteral stent may again be considered.
- However, in patients with ileal conduits or neobladders, nephroureteral catheters should not be capped because mucus produced by the bowel quickly occludes the distal sideholes, causing obstruction of a colonized system that results in infection.

Further Reading

Stokes, LS, Meranze SG. Percutaneous nephrostomy, cystostomy and nephroureteral stenting. In: Mauro MA, Murphy KPJ, Thomson KR, Venbrux AC, and Morgan RA, eds, *Image-Guided Interventions*. Philadelphia, PA: Elsevier Saunders, 2014:1076–1088.

History

▶ A 65-Year-Old Female with Cervical Cancer Status post Radiation Therapy with Leakage of Urine from Rectum

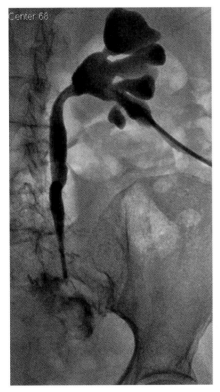

Figure 51.1

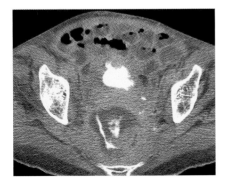

Figure 51.2

Case 51　Uretero-colic Fistula Treated with Urinary Diversion and Ureteral Embolization

Figure 51.3

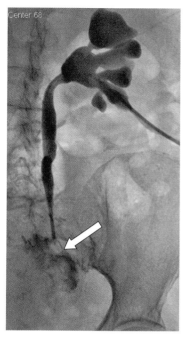

Figure 51.4

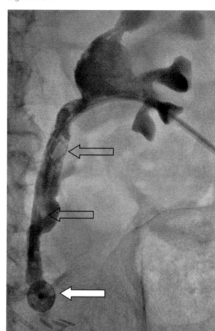

Figure 51.5

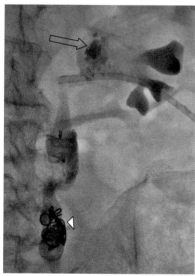

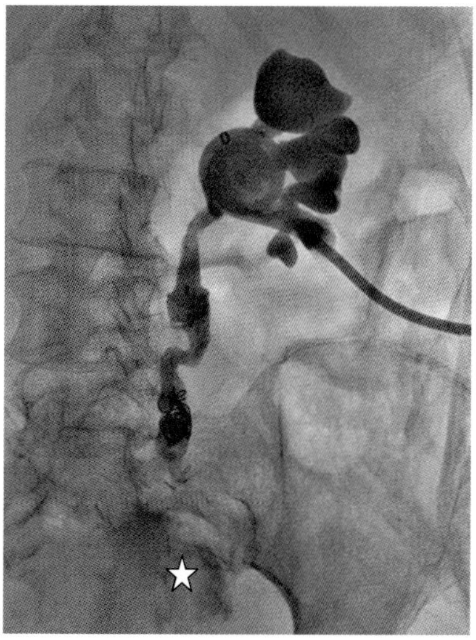

Figure 51.6

Findings

▶ Contrast injection through a right nephrostomy (Fig. 51.3) shows fistula between the ureter into an ill-defined structure at the level of the sacrum (arrow). This finding was also demonstrated by delayed imaging during a preceding contrast-enhanced computed tomography (CT) (Fig. 51.2).

- An Amplatzer vascular plug has been placed in the mid ureter above the leak (Fig. 51.4, arrow). N-butyl cyanoacrylate (NBCA) was injected into the Amplatzer vascular plug, and the small filling defects (hollow arrows) in the proximal ureter represent migrated NBCA fragments. Because the NBCA did not remain in position, additional coils were placed immediately proximal to the Amplatzer vascular plug (Fig. 51.5, arrowhead).
- After injection of Gelfoam slurry into the ureter, a second Amplatzer vascular plug was placed in the proximal ureter to complete the embolization using a "sandwich" technique (Fig. 51.5). Note residual opacified NBCA fragment in renal pelvis (hollow arrow).
- Final contrast injection into the nephrostomy demonstrates occlusion of the ureter with no evidence of leakage into the bowel (contrast overlying the pelvic brim remains from an earlier injection [Fig. 51.6, star]).

Teaching Points

- Percutaneous nephrostomy alone may be used to divert urine from ureteral or bladder fistulae. In most cases, this alone will resolve symptoms. In refractory cases, "permanent" irreversible occlusion by ureteral embolization may be required.
- Because urine contains urokinase (an anticoagulant) and does not contain blood with its associated coagulation factors, it does not clot and it can be difficult to achieve complete and durable occlusion.
- NBCA polymerizes when in contact with ionic solution. Therefore, the catheter through which it is introduced should be flushed with water (not saline) prior to injection to prevent it from solidifying within the catheter. The volume to be injected is typically estimated by a contrast injection before administration. NBCA is typically mixed with either lipiodol or tantalum powder to render it radio-opaque prior to administration. Varying concentrations of lipiodol: NBCA may be used to change the rate of polymerization, depending on the indication and location to be embolized.

Management

- There are several techniques to perform ureteral embolization. Detachable silicone balloons (not currently available in the United States) have historically provided the most durable results. Another common technique is the use of either Amplatzer vascular plugs and/or coils in conjunction with gelfoam or NBCA in a sandwich technique described in this case.

Further Reading

Schild, HH, Meyer C, Mohlenbroch M, et al. Transrenal ureter occlusion with an Amplatzer vascular plug. *J Vasc Interv Radiol.* 2009:1390–1392.

History

▶ Recurrent Ascites after Resection of Testicular Carcinoma. What Device has been Placed to Treat the Ascites?

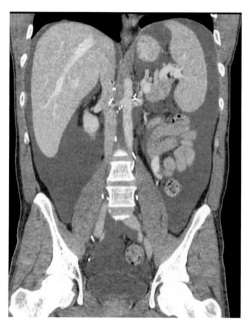

Figure 52.1

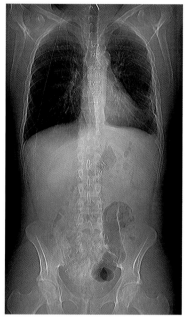

Figure 52.2

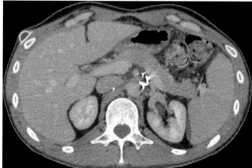

Figure 52.3

Case 52 Peritoneovenous Shunt Placement for Chylous Ascites

Figure 52.4

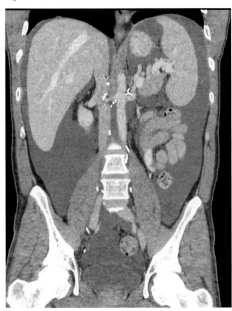

Figure 52.5

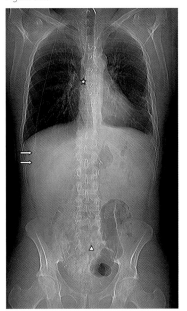

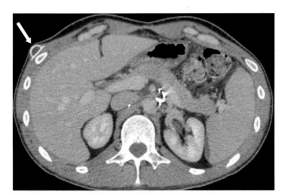

Figure 52.6

Findings

▶ Coronol computed tomography (CT) reconstruction (Fig. 52.4) shows ascites and surgical clips in the retroperitoneum suggesting previous lymph node dissection.

▶ Scout image from an abdominal CT (done for other reasons) after peritoneovenous shunt placement (Fig. 52.5) shows a contiguous catheter extending from the pelvis (arrowhead) in a subcutaneous tunnel and terminating at the high right atrium (star.) The valve (arrow) is positioned over the lower ribs.

▶ A single image from a CT 6 months after shunt placement (Fig. 52.6) shows resolution of ascites. The valve (arrow) of the shunt is seen in cross section over the lower anterolateral rib cage.

Teaching Points

▶ For select patients with refractory malignant, hepatic or chylous ascites placement of a peritoneovenous shunt can provide relief from asictes while preventing the loss of protein-rich ascites from repeated large-volume paracentesis. This procedure is most appropriate for patients with life expectancy greater than 3 months.

▶ The Denver Shunt® (Carefusion, Waukegan, IL), currently available in the United States, comes in two sizes, 11.5 F and 15.5 F, with either a double- or single-valve system. The valve prevents blood from the venous limb from back-bleeding into the ascites. The single valve is preferred for viscous or very large-volume ascites.

▶ Contraindications to shunt placement include peritonitis/sepsis, uncorrected coagulopathy, and loculated ascites. Congestive heart failure and varices are relative contraindications, as they can be aggravated by the resulting increase in intravascular volume.

Management

▶ Major complications of peritoneovenous shunt placement include disseminated intravascular coagulopathy and bacterial peritonitis. Increase in intravascular volume may aggrevate congestive heart failure and increase the risk of variceal bleeding in patients with portal hypertension.

▶ The valve chamber should be positioned over a lower chest wall for ease of access. The patient or care partner needs to pump this chamber several times a day in the supine position to prevent occlusion of the valve with protenacious or crystalloid debris.

▶ Shunts should be ligated or removed prior to abdominal surgery to prevent air in the abdomen from entering the venous system and causing air embolism.

Further Reading

Martin LG. Percutaneous placement and management of peritoneovenous shunts. *Semin Intervent Radiol.* 2012; 29(2):129–134.

History

▶ Esophageal Cancer Post Gastric Pull-up with Proximal Small-Bowel Obstruction Access for Enteral Feeding Is Required

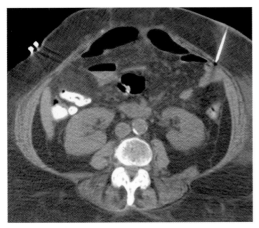

Figure 53.1

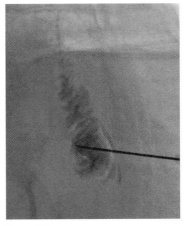

Figure 53.2

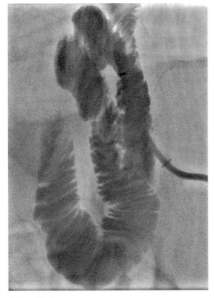

Figure 53.3

Case 53 Percutaneous Jejunostomy Catheter Placement

Figure 53.4

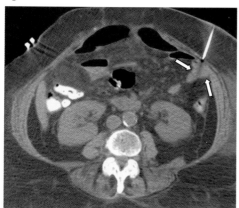

Figure 53.5

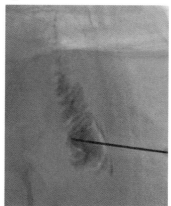

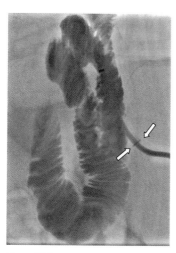

Figure 53.6

Findings

▶ Using computed tomography (CT) guidance, an 18-gauge needle has been advanced through the skin directed at a loop of decompressed small bowel in the left upper quadrant (arrows, Fig. 53.4). After the needle was advanced into the loop, contrast injection under fluoroscopy confirms intraluminal position of the needle tip (Fig. 53.5).

▶ After placement of a single retention suture (arrows, Fig. 53.6) a 12 French catheter is seen positioned within the lumen of the jejunum. Contrast injected into the catheter flows antegrade into the unobstructed more distal small bowel.

Teaching Points

▶ Compared to parenteral nutrition, enteral feeding is associated with decreased morbidity, infection, and organ failure.

▶ Percutaneous jejunostomy is indicated for enteral feeding in patients in whom the stomach is inaccessible, who have altered gastric anatomy, and/or have malignant small-bowel obstruction requiring decompression. Alternative options include endoscopic or surgical jejunostomy.

▶ CT or fluoroscopy is most commonly used to access the small bowel. When fluoroscopy is used, insufflation of the small bowel via a naso-jejunal catheter with air may be helpful to identify and distend an appropiate loop for access. An alternative method is use of ultrasound for puncture after instillation of saline into the small bowel.

▶ Access in patients with malignant bowel obstruction is less technically challanging because the target is dilated rather than decompressed. Malignant small-bowel obstruction is most commonly related to peritoneal carcinomatosis from ovarian or colon cancer.

Management

▶ In patients who have had prior jejunostomy catheters, the previously catheterized loop is usually adherent to the anterior abdominal wall and will be easier to access than a freely mobile loop.

▶ Placement of at least one anchor is helpful to promote pexy to the anterior abdominal wall and to fix the bowel to facilitate tract dilation and catheter placement.

▶ Procedure risks include peritonitis, catheter dislodgement, pericatheter leakage, and wound infection.

Further Reading

Kim YJ, Yoon CJ, Seong NJ, et al. Safety and efficacy of radiological percutaneous jejunostomy for decompression of malignant small bowel obstruction. *Eur Radiol.* 2013; *23*(10):2747–2753.

Yi F, Ge L, Zhao J, et al. Meta-analysis: total parenteral nutrition versus total enteral nutrition in predicted severe acute pancreatitis. *Intern Med.* 2012; *51*(6):523–530.

▶ Ovarian Carcinoma (Malignant Large-Bowel Obstruction)

Figure 54.4 was taken 5 days after the procedure shown in Figures 54.1–54.3.

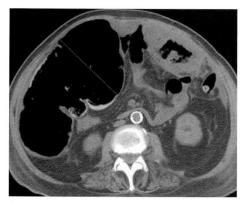

Figure 54.1

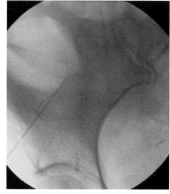

Figure 54.2

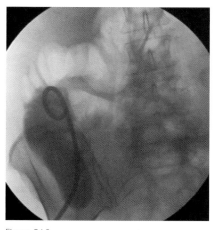

Figure 54.3

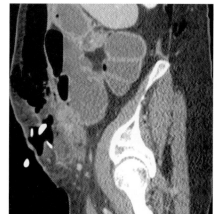

Figure 54.4

Case 54 Percutaneous Cecostomy Catheter Placement

Figure 54.5

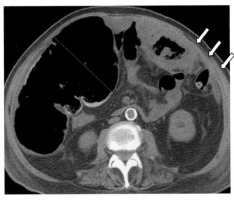

Figure 54.6

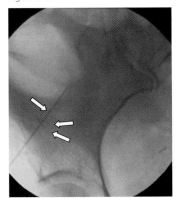

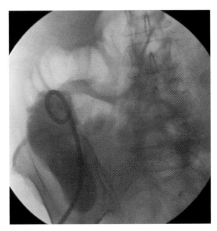

Figure 54.7

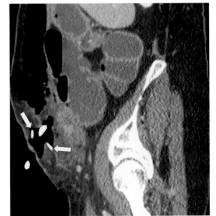

Figure 54.8

Findings

▶ Transverse diameter of the right colon in a patient with peritoneal carcinomatosis secondary to ovarian carcinoma (arrows) and distal obstruction measures 11 cm (Fig. 54.5).

▶ Three retention sutures (Fig. 54.6, arrows) have been placed to fix the mobile cecum to the anterior abdominal wall prior to catheter placement. An 18-gauge needle has been advanced between the retention sutures into the cecum.

▶ A 16 French drainage catheter has been placed into the cecum (Fig. 54.7). Contrast injection confirms intraluminal position. Note the colon is immediately decompressed after catheter placement.

▶ Sagittal reconstruction from a pelvic computed tomography (CT) scan 5 days later (Fig. 54.8) when the patient presented with cellulitis and sepsis shows extensive subcutaneous emphysema. Two of the retention suture bumpers are seen within the subcutaneous air (arrows). The other radio-opacity traversing the air represents the cecostomy catheter.

Teaching Points

▶ Retention sutures are commonly used when a catheter is placed in a mobile viscous within the abdomen (e.g., push-type gastrostomy, cecostomy, percutaneous jejunostomy). Analagous to a "buried bumper," when there is tension on retention sutures, they can invaginate into the subcutaneous tissues.

- Indications for cecostomy placment includes diversion of fecal stream in incontinent children with neurologic disorders (e.g., spina bifida, paralysis) and mechanical or pseudo-obstruction of the large bowel.
- Acute colonic distension greater than 10-12 cm is considered a risk factor for perforation.

Management

- Cecostomy to treat mechanical or pseudo-obstruction is most effective when the catheter is placed into gas within the colon rather than stool, as the latter is difficult to drain through a catheter. Because most of the drainage is gaseous, small holes should be made in the drainage collection system so that the bag does not become distended, preventing adequate drainage.
- Surgical intervention to treat malignant bowel obstruction is associated with high morbidity and mortality, up to 42% and 32%, respectively. Patients with carcinomatosis, ascites, and multilevel obstruction are unlikely to benefit from surgery for obstruction.

Further Reading

Feuer DJ, Broadley KE, Shepherd JH, et al. Surgery for the resolution of symptoms in malignant bowel obstruction in advanced gynaecological and gastrointestinal cancer. *Cochrane Database Syst Rev.* 2000; (4):CD002764.

History

▶ Squamous Cell Carcinoma of the Tongue, Gastrostomy Tube Was Requested for Enteral Feeds. What Procedure is Being Performed?

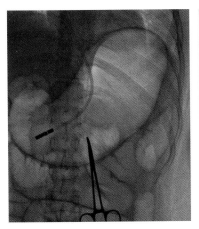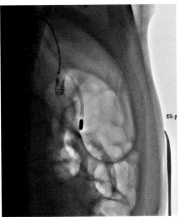

Figure 55.1

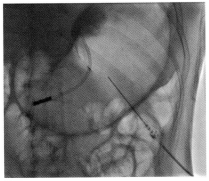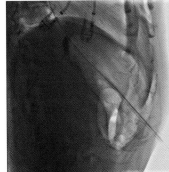

Figure 55.2

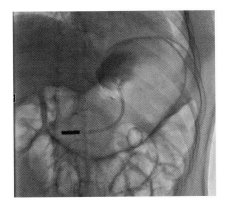

Figure 55.3

Case 55 Percutaneous Pull-through Gastrostomy

Figure 55.4

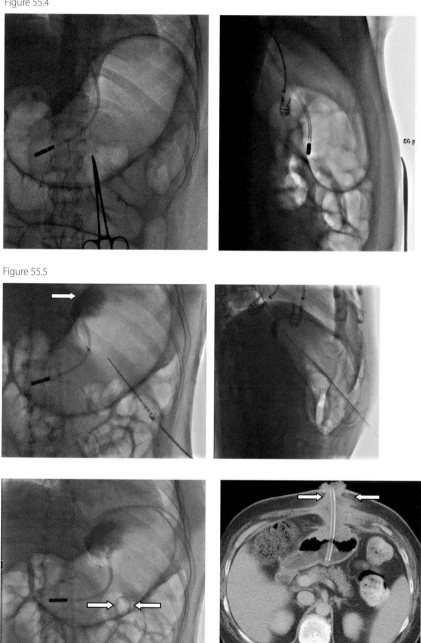

Figure 55.5

Figure 55.6

Figure 55.7

Findings

▸ Anteroposterior and lateral spot films after air insufflation via nasogastric tube (Fig. 55.4) show a distended air-filled stomach anterior to loops of small and large bowel.

▸ An 18-gauge needle attached to a contrast syringe has been advanced into the body of the stomach (Fig. 55.5). Contrast injected is seen pooling in the fundus (arrow).

▸ A wire has been manipulated from the stomach up the esophagus and out of the mouth (Fig. 55.5 lateral) to snare the 24 French gastrostomy tube, which was then pulled though the mouth and positioned with the retention bulb (arrows, Fig. 55.6) in the body of the stomach.

▸ Computed tomography (CT) 6 months after catheter placement (Fig. 55.7) shows tumor seeding the skin at the site of the gastrostomy tube (arrows).

Teaching Points

▸ Percutaneous gastrostomy may be performed by "pull-through" technique, in which through-and-through access is obtained from the anterior abdominal wall out of the mouth and the catheter is pulled through the mouth to its final position in the stomach. "Push-type" gastrostomy refers to a catheter placed directly through the abdominal wall into the stomach. Push type is often performed in conjunction with percutaneous gastropexy.

▸ For patients at high risk for gastroesophageal reflux and aspiration, transgastric jejunostomy catheters may be safer because feeds enter the gastrointestinal tract at or distal to the ligament of Treitz minimizing the liklihood of reflux. For patients who require both gastric drainage and enteral feeds, a double-bore catheter with lumina in both the stomach and a jejenum is also available.

▸ Using the pull-through technique, large-bore catheters (20–28 French) may be placed in patients who require gastric decompression. The large size of these catheters allows for drainage of a limited oral diet, which can contribute to quality of life.

▸ An unusual complication of pull-through gastrostomy is tumor implantation at the tube site. This is most common in patients with untreated squamous cell carcinoma of the head and neck or gastric cancer.

Management

▸ Preliminary ultrasound may be performed to identify the left hemiliver to avoid transhepatic catheter placement. Some operators give oral contrast the day before to opacify bowel to prevent perforation at the time of the procedure.

▸ Immediately after placement there is often a period of gastroparesis related to the procedure. Feeding may safely be started 12–24 hours after placement.

▸ Because it is not uncommon to be asked to convert a feeding gastrostomy catheter to transgastric jejunostomy catheter, the initial puncture should be made with this in mind. A direct anterior puncture into the antrum, for example, would make this conversion very difficult and catheter position tenuous.

▸ Use of prophylactic antibiotics is recommended for pull-through gastrostomy and controversial for push-type catheters.

Further Reading

Covarrubias DA, O'Connor OJ, McDermott S, et al. Radiologic percutaneous gastrostomy: review of potential complications and approach to managing the unexpected outcome. *Am J Roentgenol*. 2013; 200(4):921–931.

Yang Y, Schneider J, Düber C, et al.Comparison of fluoroscopy-guided Pull-type percutaneous radiological gastrostomy (Pull-type-PRG) with conventional percutaneous radiological gastrostomy (Push-type-PRG): clinical results in 253 patients. *Eur Radiol*. 2011; 21(11):2354–2361.

History

▶ A 63-Year-Old Female with Ovarian Cancer and Abdominal Distension

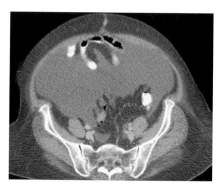

Figure 56.1

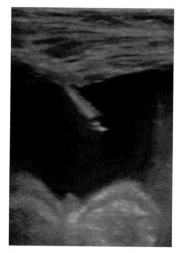

Figure 56.2

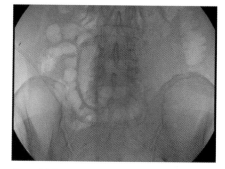

Figure 56.3

Case 56 Tunneled Drainage Placement for Relief of Recurrent Ascites

Figure 56.4

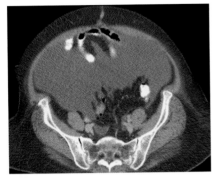

Figure 56.5

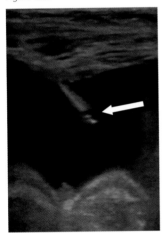

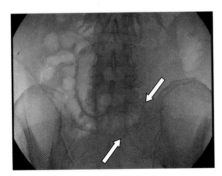

Figure 56.6

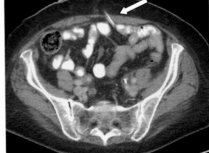

Figure 56.7

Findings

▶ Single computed tomography (CT) image (Fig. 56.4) shows marked ascites with centralization of the bowel loops in the pelvis.

▶ Ultrasound at the time of tunneled peritoneal drainage catheter placement (Fig. 56.5) shows free-flowing ascites without loculation. An 18-gauge needle (arrow) has been advanced into the ascites in the midline pelvis.

- A tunneled, multi-sidehole catheter (Fig. 56.6, arrows) was placed into the dependent pelvic ascites to provide access for intermittent drainage.
- Six weeks after placement, CT (Fig. 56.7) demonstrates good control of the ascites. The catheter is seen traversing the soft tissue of the anterior abdominal wall (arrow).

Teaching Points

- Malignant ascites is common in patients with gastric, colon, endometrial, ovarian, pancreatic, and breast cancers, lymphoma, and mesothelioma. With most tumor types, prognosis is poor, with life expectancy measured in weeks to months.
- Symptoms include abdominal distention and discomfort, shortness of breath, pain, nausea, loss of appetite, early satiety, and reduced mobility, which can significantly decrease quality of life.
- Placement of a drainage catheter allows for the patient to drain ascites intermittently at home, obviating the need for frequent hospital visits for paracentesis. This has been shown to have a positive effect on overall quality of life and symptoms, including nausea, dyspnea, and appetite loss.
- When performing paracentesis or placing a catheter, the course of the inferior epigastric arteries should be considered. Ultrasound, if available, is helpful to identify the vessels. Alternatively, midline access or an approach lateral to McBurney's point is generally safe.

Management

- Tunneled peritoneal catheters (including the Tenckhoff © shown here) with multiple sideholes are an alternative to frequent large-volume paracenteses for palliation of recurrent or malignant ascites. These are the same type of catheters typically placed surgically for peritoneal dialysis.
- In the setting of malignant ascites, diuretic therapy (typically used for nonmalignant ascites) has little role. Options for palliation generally include repeated paracentesis, nontunneled or tunneled catheter placement, and peritoneovenous shunt (see Case 52). Potential benefits of tunneled catheters compared to serial paracentesis and nontunneled catheters include stability and possibly decreased risk of infection.
- If the output decreases to less than 50 cc/drainage for three attempts over several days, and the ascites is clinically resolved, removal of the catheter should be considered.
- Complications include bacterial peritonitis, which usually necessitates removal of the catheter, catheter dislodgement, tunnel infection, and catheter blockage.

Further Reading

Akinci D, Erol B, Ciftci TT, et al. Radiologically placed tunneled peritoneal catheter in palliation of malignant ascites. *Eur J Radiol.* 2011; 80(2):265–268.

History

▶ A 68-Year-Old Male with Cholangiocarcinoma and Persistently Serum Bilirubin (Despite Endoscopic Stents) Precluding Treatment with Gemcitibine. Are there other options to maximize biliary drainage?

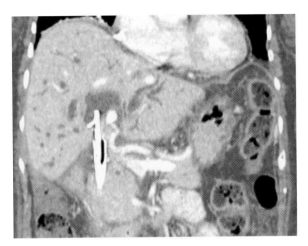

Figure 57.1

Case 57 Internal/External Biliary Drain

Figure 57.2

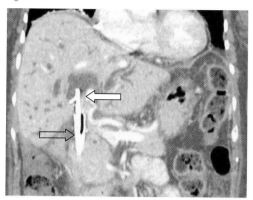

Figure 57.3

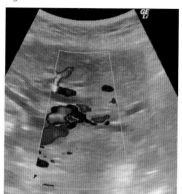

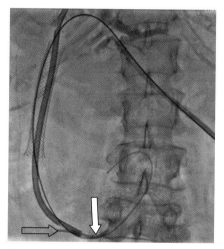

Figure 57.4

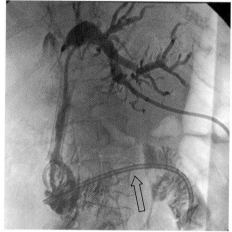

Figure 57.5

Findings

▶ Coronal computed tomography (CT) reconstruction (Fig. 57.2) shows dilated intrahepatic bile ducts despite the presence of an endoscopic plastic stent (arrow) placed through a self-expanding metallic stent (hollow arrow).

▶ Color flow ultrasound of the left hemiliver (Fig. 57.3) demonstrates dilated bile ducts adjacent to portal vein branches. Ultrasound was used to target a peripheral left bile duct.

▶ A directional catheter (arrow) has been advanced through the distal flange of the indwelling endoscopic stent (Fig. 57.4). The catheter was then advanced, thereby displacing the plastic stent into the bowel (as seen in Fig. 57.5, hollow arrow).

▶ After the endoscopic stent was removed from the biliary tree, an internal external drain was placed draining the left hemiliver (Fig. 57.4). There is effective isolation of the right biliary tree due to a near complete occlusion at the confluence of the left and right bile ducts.

Teaching Points

▶ Indications for biliary drainage include cholangitis, pruritus, biliary diversion, and lowering bilirubin for chemotherapy or palliation of other symptoms, such as anorexia.

- Endoscopic drainage is preferred in patients with low bile duct obstruction (i.e., below the confluence of the right and left hepatic ducts) because placement of a single stent will drain the entire biliary tree.
- Percutaneous biliary drainage is indicated for the treatment of high bile duct obstruction because a specific ductal system may be targeted or when endoscopic drainage of low bile duct obstruction is unsuccessful or not possible due to altered anatomy.
- The status of the portal vein, the presence of parenchymal atrophy or ascites, location of tumors, and the presence of bile duct isolation should be considered when planning biliary drainage.
- The left hepatic duct is longer than the right, and the right biliary tree is therefore more susceptible to isolation. Isolation can often be anticipated based on preprocedure cross sectional imaging (CT, magnetic resonance) but is not always accurate.
- Percutaneous biliary drainage is performed with fluoroscopic guidance. Ultrasound may be used for the initial puncture of the bile duct, and is particularly helpful in left-sided biliary drainage.
- External biliary catheters may be placed in the setting of sepsis to minimize manipulation, when the obstruction cannot be crossed, or when high output from an internal/external drain causes dehydration or electrolyte abnormalities. External biliary catheters are obligatory external drainage catheters because they are generally placed above the obstruction.
- The Bismuth-Corlette classification of hilar cholangiocarcinoma has been used to describe the extent of high bile duct obstruction:

  Type 1 involves common hepatic duct but not the confluence.

  Type 2 involves the confluence of the right and left hepatic ducts.

  Type 3 extends to involve a right or left secondary confluence.

  Type 4 involves both the right and left secondary duct confluence.

Management

- Catheter sideholes must be positioned both above and below the obstruction to provide adequate drainage. All sideholes should be in the biliary tree (or bowel) because sideholes in the tract will cause pericatheter leakage.
- Catheters should be flushed forward at least daily to retain patency. Routine exchange every 2–3 months is recommended to prevent occlusion.

Further Reading

Covey AM, Brown KT. Palliative percutaneous drainage in malignant biliary obstruction. Part 1: indications and preprocedure evaluation. *J Support Oncol.* 2006; 4(6):269–273.
Covey AM, Brown KT. Palliative percutaneous drainage in malignant biliary obstruction. Part 2: Mechanisms and postprocedure management. *J Support Oncol.* 2006; 4(7):329–335.

History

▶ Resection of Cavernous Hepatic Hemangioma Complicated by Intrahepatic Abscess, Fever, and Leukocytosis
After drainage of the abscess (Fig. 58.2) there is persistent bilious output from the catheter. What is the next step in management?

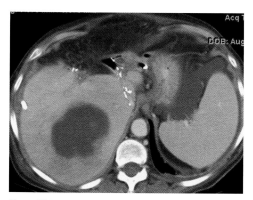

Figure 58.1

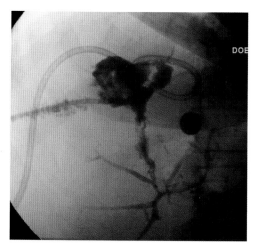

Figure 58.2

Case 58 Intrahepatic Biloma

Figure 58.3

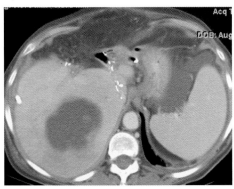

Figure 58.4

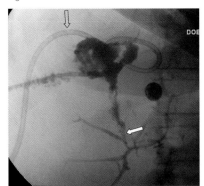

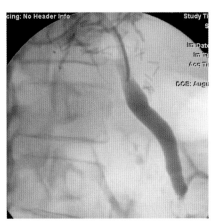

Figure 58.5

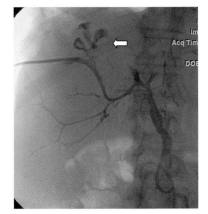

Figure 58.6

Findings

▶ Abdominal computed tomography (CT) scan demonstrates an intrahepatic collection with a thick wall in the remnant right hemiliver (Fig. 58.3). On this axial image, a small part of a perihepatic drainage catheter is seen.

▶ After percutaneous drainage of the intraheptic abscess, contrast injection into the drainage catheter (Fig. 58.4) demonstrates communication with the nondilated biliary tree (arrow). Again, note is made of the perihepatic catheter previously placed in a separate collection (hollow arrow).

▶ Two weeks after drainage of the biloma, a directional catheter was advanced from the abscess into the biliary tree (Fig. 58.5), and an internal external biliary drain (Fig. 58.6) was placed via the biloma. Additional sideholes were added to the catheter to provide ongoing decompression of the residual abscess cavity (arrow).

Teaching Points

▶ Biloma and abscess are in the differential diagnosis for intrahepatic collections after liver surgery. Bilomas occur either because of iatrogenic injury to the biliary tree or secondary to downstream obstruction.

▶ After initial decompression of the abscess cavity, a change in the character of the output from purulent to bilious confirms communication with the biliary tree.

▶ Other causes of liver abscess include hematogenous spread from gastrointestinal infection, including appendicitis and diverticulitis. Hydatid (echinococcal) cyst is also in the differential and is characterized by septae and mural calcifications.

Management

▶ Placement of any drainage catheter into the liver should be planned to avoid the pleura if possible to eliminate the risk of contamination of the chest. For collections high in the liver that contain air, access from a subcostal approach can be performed using the air as the target under fluoroscopy.

▶ Patients should be pretreated with antibiotics prior to drainage of a liver abscess, as the risk of sepsis related to manipulation is high.

▶ Patients should be counseled that bile leaks can take several weeks to months to resolve. Bilomas may resolve with long-term catheter drainage, but may require diversion of the bile ducts with either percutaneous or endoscopic drainage. Occasionally, as in this case, effective drainage of both the infected biloma and the biliary tree may be achieved from a single access.

Further Reading

Brown KT, Covey AM. Management of malignant biliary obstruction. *Tech Vasc Interv Radiol.* 2008; 11(1):43–50.

History

▶ Cholangiocarcinoma With Intractable Pruritus. Based on the Cholangiogram in Figure 59.2, What is the Optimal Treatment Strategy for This Patient?

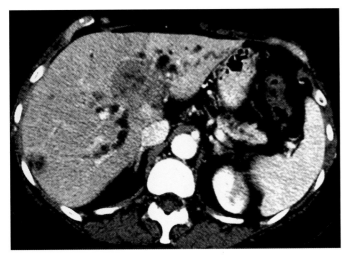

Figure 59.1

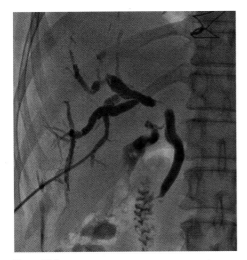

Figure 59.2

Case 59 Primary Biliary Stent

Figure 59.3

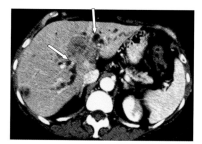

Figure 59.4

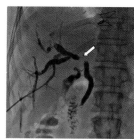

Figure 59.5

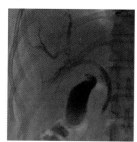

Findings

▶ Figure 59.3 is a single image from a contrast-enhanced computed tomography (CT) showing a central liver mass and dilation of the intrahepatic bile ducts. Both the right and left (arrows) hepatic ducts appear to converge on the mass, suggesting they are isolated from each other.

▶ Percutaneous cholangiogram from a right posterior approach shows a short-segment, high-grade obstruction of the right hepatic duct (arrow, Fig. 59.4). Note there is no filling of left-sided ducts or the right anterior ducts, representing complete isolation of the right posterior bile ducts.

▶ A self-expanding metallic stent (SEMS) has been placed across the obstruction, allowing internal drainage of the right posterior bile ducts, reestablishing enterohepatic circulation of bile (Fig. 59.5).

Teaching Points

▶ Effective drainage of a single liver segment will most often relieve the symptom of pruritus.

▶ It is critical to obtain high-quality cross sectional imaging to appropriately plan for biliary intervention. Attention should be taken to assess for any bile duct isolation, liver atrophy, the presence of ascites, and tumor location.

▶ When ductal systems are completely isolated, as in this case, the risk of contaminating the nonvisualized bile ducts is very low. When bile ducts that are not adequately drained fill with contrast, cholangitis is common.

▶ The mean patency of uncovered SEMS in the biliary tree is 6–9 months, and once placed, they cannot be removed. Therefore, they are used most often to treat malignant bile duct obstruction.

▶ Stents placed across the papilla allow reflux of small-bowel contents into the biliary tree while the stent is patent. In this situation, if/when the stent occludes in the future patients often present with cholangitis due to obstruction of the contaminated biliary tree. When the stent can be placed above the papilla, as in this case, integrity of the sphincter and sterility of the biliary tree are maintained making the chance of cholangitis in the future low.

▶ To treat malignant biliary obstruction in the absence of cholangitis, stent placement is often the best option to minimize catheter-related complications, such as leaking, dislodgment, and the care that an exteriorized device requires.

Management

▶ Placement of the stent effectively converts high bile duct obstruction to a situation that can be managed endoscopically in the future if/when the stent occludes.

▶ When placed primarilary or within 1–2 weeks after initial drainage, plugging of the access tract with gelfoam may decrease the risk of bile leaking into the peritoneum.

Further Reading

Brown KT, Covey AM. Management of malignant biliary obstruction. *Tech Vasc Interv Radiol.* 2008;11(1):43–50.

Thornton RH, Frank BS, Covey AM, et al. Catheter-free survival after primary percutaneous stenting of malignant bile duct obstruction. *Am J Roentgenol.* 2011; 197(3):W514–8.

History

▶ Pancreatic Cancer With Right Upper Quadrant Pain, Fever, and Leukocytosis 10 Days after Endoscopic Stent Placement. What is the Diagnosis?

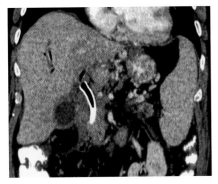

Figure 60.1

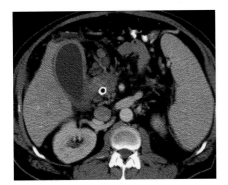

Figure 60.2

Case 60 Biliary Stent Complicated by Cholecystitis

Figure 60.3

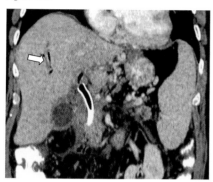

Figure 60.4

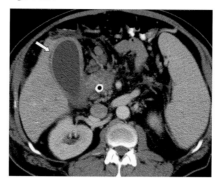

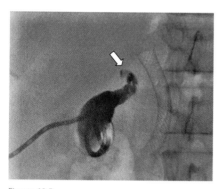

Figure 60.5

Findings

▶ Coronal reconstruction and axial image from a contrast enhanced CT shows a metallic biliary stent in the common hepatic duct (Figs. 60.3 and 60.4). There is air in the intrahepatic bile ducts (Fig. 60.3, arrow), which are nondilated, suggesting the stent is patent.

▶ The gallbladder (Fig. 60.4, arrow) is distended and thick walled with mural low density, suggesting gallbladder wall edema. These findings are consistent with acute cholecystitis.

▶ In Figure 60.5, a percutaneous cholecystostomy catheter has been placed. Contrast injection after decompression shows an intact gallbladder. The proximal cystic duct is identified (arrow), but no contrast is seen passing into the common hepatic duct. No intraluminal stones are identified.

Teaching Points

▶ Placement of even a bare (i.e., noncovered) metallic stent across the insertion of the cystic duct is complicated by acute cholecystitis in a minority of patients. Similarly, stent placement across the pancreatic duct can result in pancreatitis.

▶ Covered stents are more likely to result in cholangitis and pancreatitis, but to date there is no clear evidence of improved patency compared to bare stents.

▶ Contrast injection at the time of initial cholecystostomy should only replace the volume of bile drained. Overdistension of the gallbladder with contrast should be avoided to minimize the risk of sepsis secondary to bacterial translocation.

▶ Percutaneous cholecystostomy is used to treat acalculous cholecystitis or for patients with calculus cholecystitis who are poor candidates for operation due to comorbidities.

- Occasionally a cholecystostomy catheter may be used to provide biliary drainage in the setting of low bile duct obstruction if the obstruction is below the cystic duct insertion when percutaneous biliary drainage is not feasible.

Management

- Antibiotics should be given within 1 hour of drainage of an abdominal abscess to minimize the risk of sepsis.
- Removal of a cholecystostomy catheter requires (1) formation of a tract between the gallbladder and skin to prevent leakage of bile into the peritoneum, which usually occurs in 4–6 weeks and (2) re-establishment of patency of the cystic duct. Alternatively, these may be lifelong catheters, as in this patient with metastatic pancreatic cancer, or can be removed at the time of cholecystectomy.
- The character and volume of output is helpful in management. Typically there is little output as long as the cystic duct is occluded. Increase in volume of bilious output is indicative of cystic duct patency.

Further Reading

Ginat D, Saad WE. Cholecystostomy and transcholecystic biliary access. *Tech Vasc Interv Radiol.* 2008; 11(1):2–13.

Shimizu S, Naitoh I, Nakazawa T, et al. Predictive factors for pancreatitis and cholecystitis in endoscopic covered metal stenting for distal malignant biliary obstruction. *J Gastroenterol Hepatol.* 2013; 28(1):68–72.

History

▶ Colon Cancer Status Post Biliary Wall Stent Placement 4 Months Ago Presents with Fever and Leukocytosis

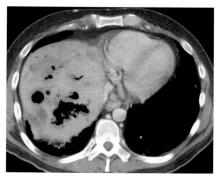

Figure 61.1

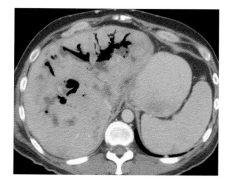

Figure 61.2

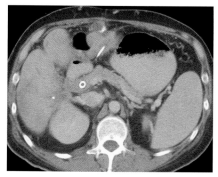

Figure 61.3

Case 61 Occluded Wall Stent Complicated by Cholangitis and Cholangitic Abscesses

Figure 61.4

Figure 61.5

Figure 61.6

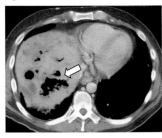

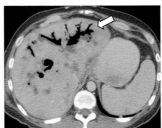

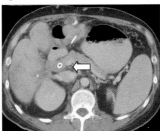

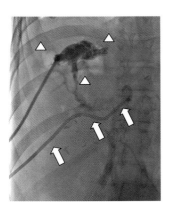

Figure 61.7

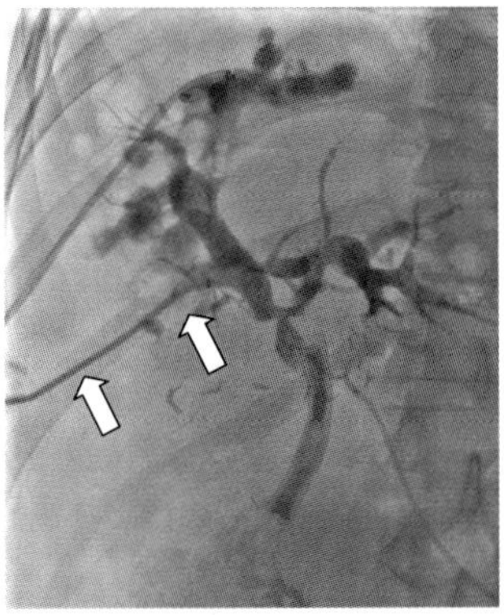

Figure 61.8

Findings

▸ A predominantly air-filled cholangitic abscess is seen in segment 7 (arrow, Fig. 61.4).

▸ Figure 61.5 shows the intrahepatic bile ducts are markedly dilated with gas and contain gas-fluid levels (arrow) consistent with biliary obstruction. A metallic biliary stent (arrow) is seen in Figure 61.6.

▸ Figure 61.7 is an image from the placement of a right-to-left external biliary drainage catheter (arrows), At the same sitting an abscess drain was placed into the cholangitic abscess that is opacified with both air and injected contrast (arrowheads). Contrast injected into the abscess catheter (Fig. 61.8) confirms communication with the biliary tree.

Teaching Points

▸ Cholangitis almost always occurs in the setting of a colonized biliary tree. Bacterial colonization may result from previous bilioenteric anastamosis, sphincterotomy, or indwelling stent placed across the papilla, as in this case.

▸ After initial drainage of purulent material from the abscess, a change in character of the output to bile confirms communication with the biliary tree.

▸ Simply identifying gas in the biliary tree in a patient with a stent or bilioenteric bypass does not confirm adequate drainage. Bile ducts overdistended with gas may also be a sign of occlusion.

▸ Bile ducts are not always dilated in the setting of a cholangitic abscess because the abscess can decompress the obstructed biliary tree (see Case 58).

▸ The two most common causes of liver abscesses are gastrointestinal infection (appendicitis or diverticulitis) and biliary obstruction.

Management

▶ Cholangitic abscesses are a result of obstruction of a contaminated biliary tree.

▶ Drainage of the abscess is usually sufficient to temporize a septic patient. Definitive treatment requires relief of biliary obstruction which, depending on the level of obstruction, may be achieved percutaneously, endoscopically, or, less commonly, surgically.

Further Reading

Brown KT, Covey AM. Management of malignant biliary obstruction. *Tech Vasc Interv Radiol.* 2008; 11(1):43–50.

Case 62

History

▸ A 72-Year-Old Male with Right Lower-Extremity Progressive Leg Heaviness and Pain Presents with the Following Clinical Findings and Ultrasound

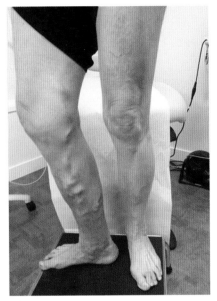

Figure 62.1

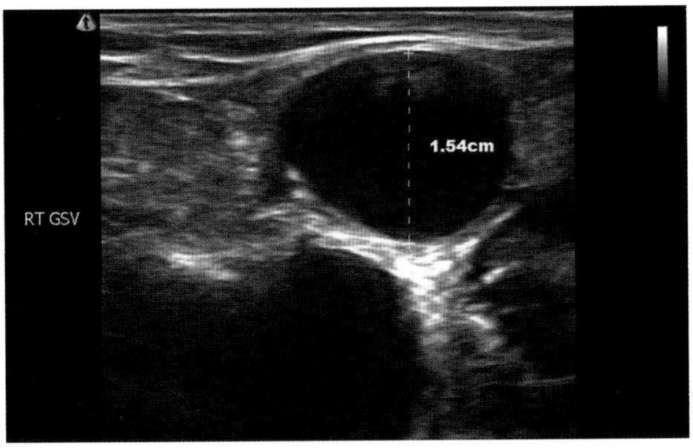

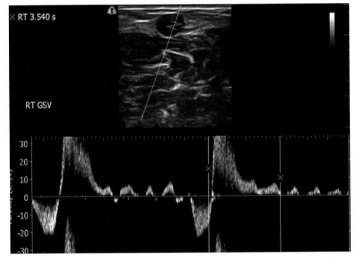

Figure 62.2

Figure 62.3

Case 62 Varicose Veins—Greater Saphenous Vein Reflux

Figure 62.4

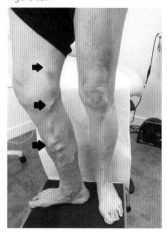

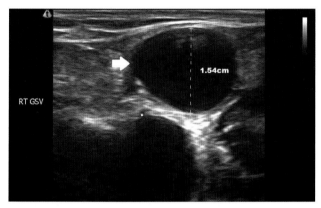

Figure 62.5

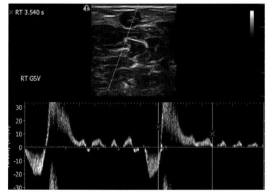

Figure 62.6

Findings

▸ Figure 62.4 demonstrate dilated varicose veins in the greater saphenous distribution (arrows).

▸ Figure 62.5 show the dilated greater saphenous vein (arrow) measuring up to 1.54 cm.

▸ Figure 62.6 demonstrates reversal of flow within this vein during calf compression maneuvers.

Teaching Points

▶ Physical examination should include color photographs, pulse checks, a search for ulcers, and skin changes. Often dilated veins in certain territories suggest certain reflux patterns.

▶ Grayscale and duplex ultrasound evaluation should be performed with the patient standing. Evaluation should include:
  - Deep and superficial vein patency
  - Maximal diameter of the abnormal vein (normal GSV <4 mm and normal SSV <3 mm)
  - Measure minimal skin depth to vein
  - Document tortuosity
  - Search for reflux of saphenous veins and tributaries
  - Document any perforator larger than 3–4 mm and evaluate for incompetence

▶ If the vein to be ablated is less than 1 cm from the skin, the risk of skin burn increases. Careful tumescent placement may reduce this risk.

▶ Tumescent fluid administration should be delivered under direct ultrasound guidance with the objective of shielding the target vein from the surrounding tissues and to collapse the vein against the ablation device to allow for maximal contact.

▶ Maximal tolerated doses of lidocaine are 4.5 mg/kg of lidocaine without epinephrine and 7 mg/kg with epinephrine.

▶ Tumescent concentration usually ranges from 0.05% to 0.1% lidocaine. For a 45 cm treatment segment, a volume of 100–150 cc of 0.1% lidocaine is usually sufficient.

Management

▶ Treatment for saphenous vein involves endovenous ablation therapy. Treatment with endovenous therapy should be reserved for symptomatic patients with reflux.

▶ After recovery for endovenous ablative therapy, residual disease may be treated with sclerotherapy or a combination of sclerotherapy and microphelbectomy.

Acknowledgments

Images courtesy of Neil M. Khilnani, MD, Weill Cornell Medical College, New York, NY.

Further Reading

Gloviczki P, Gloviczki ML. Guidelines for the management of varicose veins. *Phlebology* 2012; 27:s2–s9. Min R, Khilnani N. Endovenous laser ablation of varicose veins. *J Cardiovasc Surg.* 2005; 46:395–405.

History

▶ A 59-Year-Old Male with Hepatitis C, Cirrhosis, and Bleeding Esophageal Varices with Failure of Banding

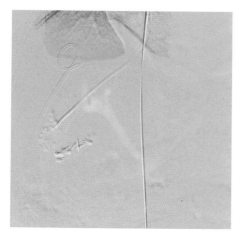

Figure 63.1

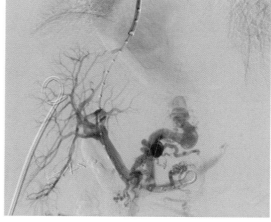

Figure 63.2

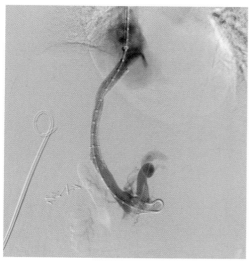

Figure 63.3

Case 63 Transjugular Intrahepatic Portosystemic Shunt

Figure 63.4

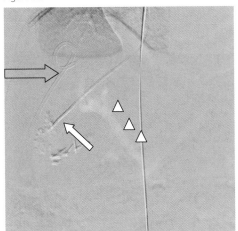

Figure 63.4

Figure 63.5

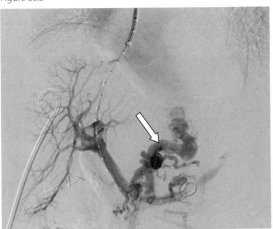

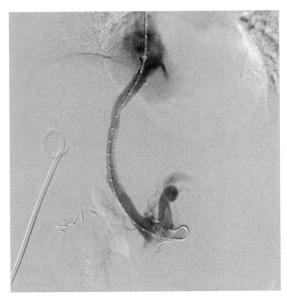

Figure 63.6

Findings

► Wedged CO_2 venography (Fig. 63.4) with a catheter in the right hepatic vein (arrow) is shown to delineate the position of the portal vein (arrowheads) in relation to the hepatic vein and to provide a target for transhepatic portal venous puncture. A pigtail drainage catheter to treat refractory ascites is seen in the right upper quadrant (hollow arrow).

► After successful portal vein access has been achieved, venogram with the catheter positioned in the central splenic vein (arrow, Fig. 63.5) demonstrates enlarged left gastric (coronary) and epigastric varices (arrow).

► After transjugular intrahepatic portosystemic shunt (TIPS) creation with a covered stent extending from the confluence of the right hepatic vein/inferior vena cava to the main portal vein (Fig. 63.6), there is good flow through the TIPS and decrease in the size of the varices.

Teaching Points

▶ TIPS is indicated to treat symptoms related to portal venous hypertension, including intractable ascites, refractory bleeding from esophageal varices, and occasionally Budd-Chiari syndrome.

▶ CO_2 can be used for wedged hepatic venography because it easily crosses the capillary sinusoids from a wedged hepatic vein and provides excellent opacification of the portal vein. An occlusion balloon is used to prevent reflux of CO_2 in the hepatic vein.

▶ TIPS reduces portosystemic pressure gradient in over 90% of patients. To control variceal bleeding, a portosystemic pressure gradient of <10–12 mmHg is recommended. The pressure gradient endpoint when TIPS is used to treat refractory ascites is much debated, with most gradient endpoint recommendations being lower than that for treatment of variceal bleeding. Caution must be taken as the rate of hepatic encephalopathy increases with decreased gradients. Use of TIPS to control bleeding is more effective (~90% success) than for use in refractory ascites (70%–80% success).

▶ Covered stents are used to prevent intrastent stenosis associated with uncovered stents related to bile contamination of the TIPS. The covered portion of the stent should extend from the portal vein to the confluence of the hepatic vein and inferior vena cava.

Management

▶ Patients with Model for End Stage Liver Disease (MELD) scores over 18 have high risk of 3-month mortality.

▶ Ultrasound is the preferred method to evaluate for stent patency after placement. The first baseline study should be performed several days after placement to allow time for dissipation of air bubbles trapped in the covered portion of the stent. Shunt velocity of <50 or >200 cm/s or a change from baseline of >50 cm/s suggests shunt malfunction. After the initial Doppler study, surveillance is performed at 3 months, and every 6 months thereafter.

▶ Stenosis/occlusion at the hepatic vein end of the stent is the most common cause of failure. This can be treated with venoplasty or placement of a second stent.

▶ Reversal (coil embolization) or partial reversal (stent within a stent) may be considered when there is hepatic encephalopathy refractory to treatment or worsening liver failure due to the volume of flow bypassing the hepatic parenchyma after TIPS creation.

Further Reading

Gaba RC, Khiatani VL, Knuttinen MG, et al. Comprehensive review of TIPS technical complications and how to avoid them. *Am J Roentgenol.* 2011; 196(3):675–685.

Case 64

History

- Hematemeis. What is the Procedure Being Performed?

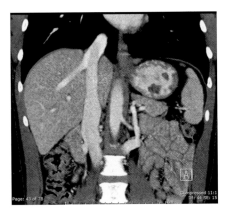

Figure 64.1

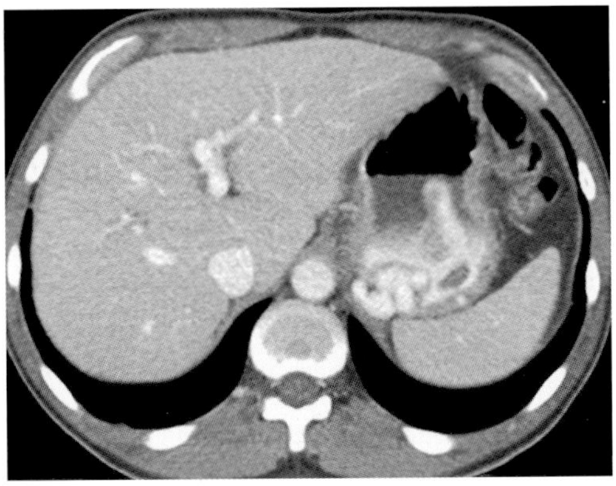

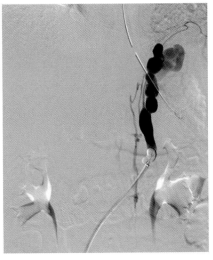

Figure 64.2

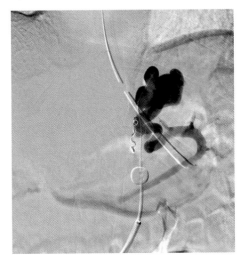

Figure 64.3

Figure 64.4

Case 64 Balloon-Occluded Retrograde Transvenous Obliteration of Gastric Varices

Figure 64.5

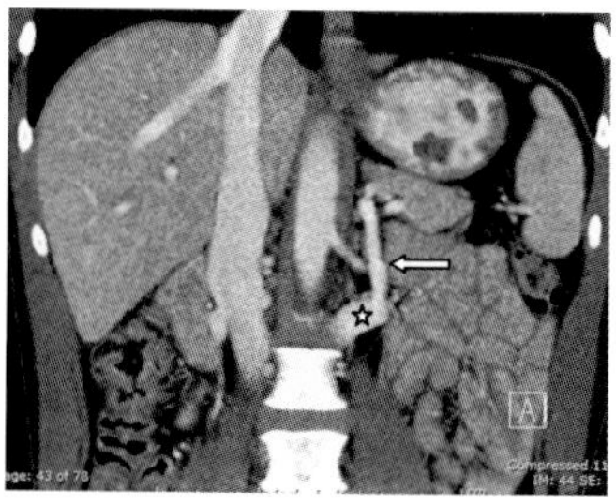

Figure 64.6

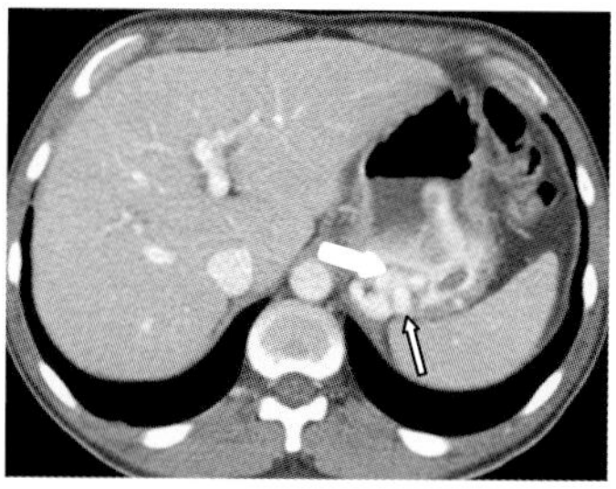

Figure 64.7

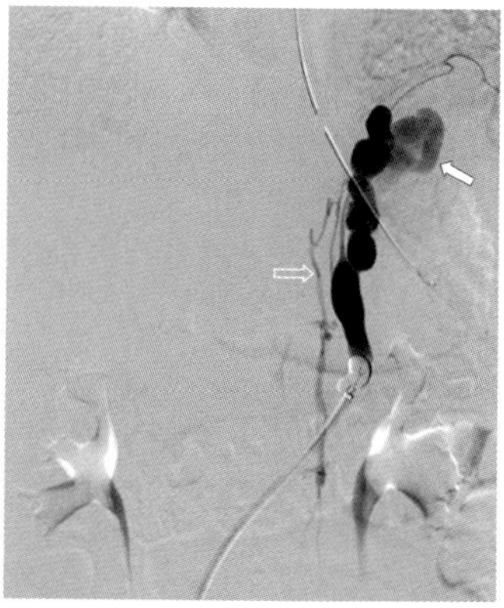

Figure 64.8

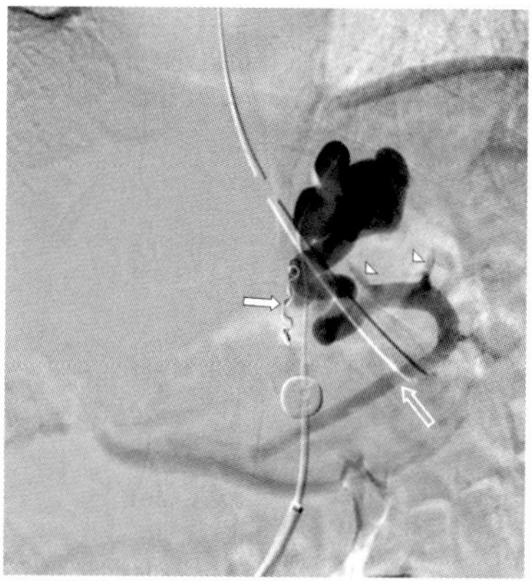

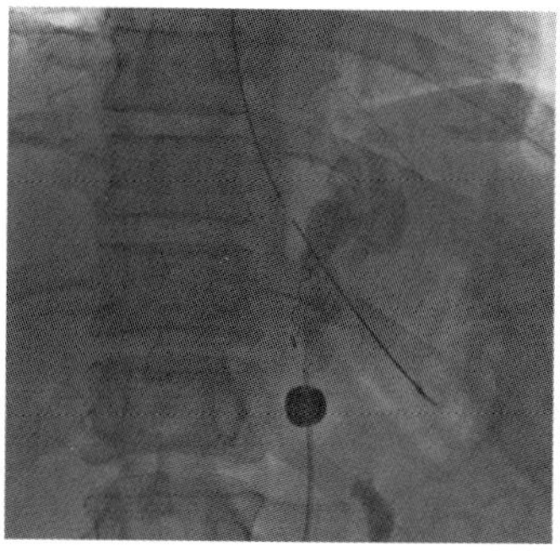

Figure 64.9

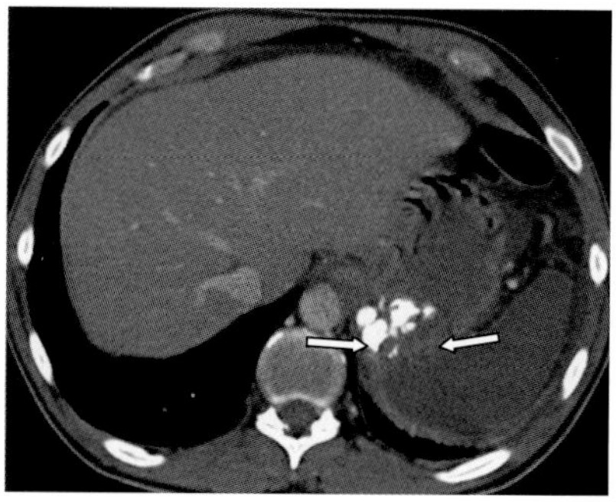

Figure 64.10

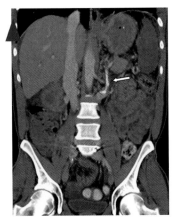

Figure 64.11

Findings

▶ A coronal reformat (Fig. 64.5) from a contrast-enhanced computed tomography (CT) demostrates a large gastrorenal shunt (arrow) arising from the left renal vein (star). An axial image from the same CT (Fig. 64.6) shows submucosal gastric varices (hollow arrow) covered by a thin layer of gastric mucosa (arrow).

▶ The gastrorenal shunt (GRS) has been catheterized from a femoral vein approach (Fig. 64.7). Contrast injection with a balloon inflated fills the gastric varices (arrow). A systemic vein (phrenic) is seen medial to the shunt (hollow arrow).

▶ After coil embolization of the systemic vein (arrow), the catheter has been advanced distally within the shunt (Fig. 64.8). Contrast injection shows reflux into short gastric veins (arrowheads) and the splenic vein (hollow arrow). Note that contrast is injected through the endhole of the catheter, and a more proximal balloon is inflated to prevent reflux.

▶ With the balloon of the catheter inflated, a sclerosant has been injected to fill the volume of the GRS and varices (Fig. 64.9).

▶ One month after balloon-occluded retrograde transvenous obliteration (BRTO), contrast-enhanced CT (Figs. 64.10 and 64.11) shows retention of lipiodol in the embolized gastric varices (arrows). There is no residual enhancement of the GRS or varices.

Teaching Points

▶ Indications for BRTO are bleeding or high-risk gastric varices and hepatic encephalopathy secondary to shunt volume. Unlike TIPS, BRTO can be performed in the setting of decompensated liver function and encephalopathy, and it may even improve encephalopathy by increasing hepatopedal flow in the portal vein.

▶ In some cases, BRTO can be performed in conjunction with TIPS or balloon-occluded antegrade transvenous obliteration (BATO) to relieve sequela of portal hypertension.

▶ The sclerosant is typically a mixture of 1 part ethiodol, 2 parts 3% sotradechol, and 3 parts air agitated through a three-way syringe into a liquid foam. The average injectate is approximately 30–50 cc.

Management

▶ The balloon of the catheter is left inflated for a 4- to 24-hour dwell time of the sclerosant to obliterate the shunt and varices.

▶ Portal vein thrombosis is a relative contraindication to BRTO because it can cause increased venous pressure in the mesenteric veins. Other potential complications include liver failure and gastric ulcers.

▶ Follow-up imaging with either CT, magnetic resonance, or endoscopic ultrasound is important to evaluate for residual varices that may require additional therapy.

Further Reading

Saad, WEA, Al-Osaimi AMS, Caldwell SH. Pre and post balloon occluded retrograde transvenous obliteration clinical evaluation, management and imaging: indications, management protocols and follow up. *Tech Vasc Interv Radiol.* 2012; 15(3):165–202.

History

▶ A 45-Year-Old Female with Uncontrolled Hypertension

A right adrenal nodule is identified on computed tomography (CT) imaging with Houndsfield value of −7. What is being shown here?

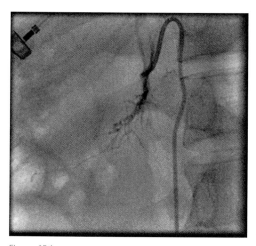

Figure 65.1

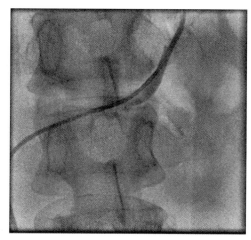

Figure 65.2

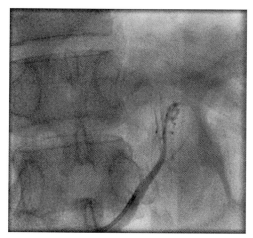

Figure 65.3

Case 65   Adrenal Vein Sampling

Figure 65.4

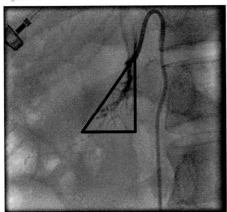

Figure 65.5

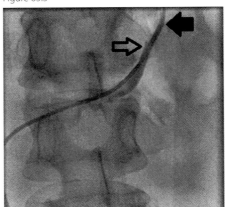

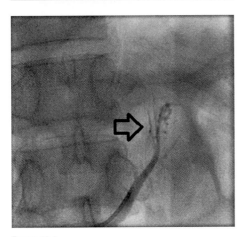

Figure 65.6

Table 65.1

			RATIO
SERUM	Aldosterone	105.8 ng/dL	4.2
	Cortisol	24.9 µg/dL	
RIGHT	Aldosterone	15,180 ng/dL	52.1
	Cortisol	291.5 µg/dL	
LEFT	Aldosterone	363 ng/dL	2.1
	Cortisol	175.45 µg/dL	

Findings

▶ The right adrenal vein has been catheterized and a small amount of contrast has been injected by hand (Fig. 65.4). The adrenal gland can be recognized angiographically as a gland-like structure, which is usually triangular in appearance (triangle).

▶ Figure 65.5 demonstrates the catheter in the left adrenal vein (hollow arrow). Reflux of contrast is noted in the left inferior phrenic vein inflow (black arrow). This is a common finding with the left adrenal vein and left inferior phrenic vein draining into a common trunk prior to joining the left renal vein.

▶ Figure 65.6 show the left adrenal gland (hollow arrow).

▶ Table 65.1 shows levels of aldosterone and cortisol in the serum, right and left adrenal veins. Elevated cortisol levels in the adrenal vein samples help to confirm that the samples are from the adrenal glands. An aldosterone to cortisol ratio in the adrenal vein that is higher than that of serum suggests unilateral hormone production from the right adrenal adenoma.

Teaching Points

▶ Adrenal vein sampling is performed to determine whether autonomous hormone production is unilateral or bilateral, thereby directing therapy.
  ▪ Most commonly performed for primary aldosteronism
  ▪ Less commonly performed to isolate biochemically proven pheochromocytoma not visible on imaging.

▶ While there are some exceptions, the drainage of the central adrenal veins is fairly constant. The right central adrenal vein typically drains into the midposterior wall of the inferior vena cava, while the left central adrenal vein usually joins the inferior phrenic before entering the left renal vein.

▶ Preprocedure computed tomography (CT) scan can be helpful in identifying the adrenal vein, expected location of the adrenal gland, and characterization of mass lesions. It should be noted that adenomas detected on CT may not necessarily be associated with the patient's clinical symptoms.

▶ Comparison of the adrenal vein blood samples and peripheral blood is performed. A cortisol level at least 2–3 times that of peripheral blood confirms accurate adrenal vein sampling.
  ▪ Adrenals producing aldosterone will show an aldosterone-cortisol ratio higher than that of the peripheral blood sample.
  ▪ Normal glands will result in a ratio that is equal to or less than peripheral blood.
  ▪ In cases of unilateral adenoma, the contralateral normal adrenal gland may show suppressed aldosterone secretion.

Management

▶ Postprocedure management includes bed rest for femoral venipuncture.

▶ In cases with persistent pain after a procedure with escalating analgesic requirements, consider intraadrenal hemorrhage as a cause.

Further Reading

Daunt N. Adrenal vein sampling: how to make it quick, easy, and successful. *Radiographics* 2005; 25:S143–S158.

History

▶ A 45-Year-Old Male with Biopsy-Proven Small Cell Carcinoma in the Right Chest Presents with Acute Shortness of Breath and Facial Swelling

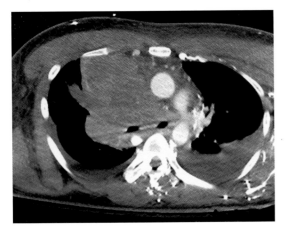

Figure 66.1

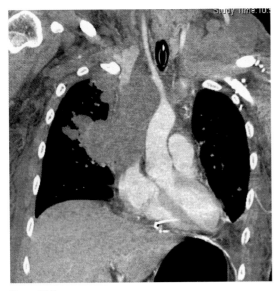

Figure 66.2

Case 66   Superior Vena Cava Syndrome

Figure 66.3

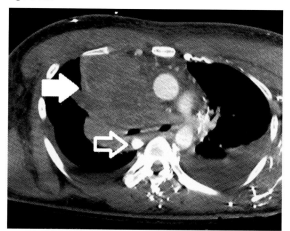

Figure 66.4

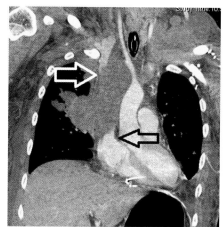

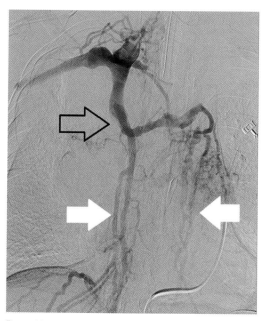

Figure 66.5

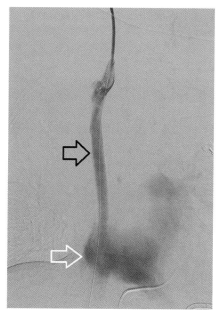

Figure 66.6

Findings

▸ A large mass is seen in the right upper lobe (Fig. 66.3) extending into the hilum (white arrow). Of note, the superior vena cava (SVC) is not identified and contrast is seen filling a dilated azygous venous system (white hollow arrow).

▸ Coronal images through the chest (Fig. 66.4) demonstrate the right upper lobe mass with complete occlusion of the SVC just distal to the confluence of the right internal jugular and subclavian veins (white hollow arrow) to the level of the mid atrium (black hollow arrow).

▸ Venogram performed from the right internal jugular vein (Fig. 66.5) demonstrates SVC occlusion (black hollow arrow) with filling of the azygous and accessory hemiazygous systems (white arrows).

▸ Placement of an SVC stent (Fig. 66.6, black arrow) demonstrates rapid transit of contrast into the right atrium (white arrow). Note that the azygous and hemiazygous systems no longer fill.

Teaching Points

▶ Symptoms of SVC syndrome include dyspnea, facial and/or upper-extremity swelling, cough, stridor, chest pain, or cyanosis.

▶ The most common cause of SVC syndrome is malignancy, with lung cancer being the most common.

▶ Benign causes of SVC syndrome include catheter-related stenosis and granulomatous mediastinitis and radiation therapy.

▶ Primary patency is 70%–80% in 6 months, with secondary patency ~95% at 6 months.

Management

▶ First-line therapy for acute malignant SVC syndrome is stenting with concomitant radiation and/or chemotherapy. Benign disease may be treated with balloon venoplasty and/or stent placement.

▶ Venous thrombolysis, either mechanical or chemical, may need to be performed prior to stenting if acute thrombus is present.

▶ Most patients experience complete resolution of symptoms within 1–3 days after stenting.

▶ Use of postprocedure anticoagulation/antiplatelet is controversial.

▶ Complications include stent migration and cardiac tamponade due to rupture of the SVC into the pericardium.

Further Reading

Ganeshan A, Hon LQ, Warakaulle DR, et al. Superior vena caval stenting for SVC obstruction: current status. *Eur J Radiol.* 2009;71:343–349.

Warren P, Burke C. Endovascular management of chronic upper extremity deep vein thrombosis and superior vena cava syndrome. *Semin Intervent Radiol.* 2011; 28:32–38.

History

▶ A 17-Year-Old Wrestler with Pain and Swelling of the Right Arm

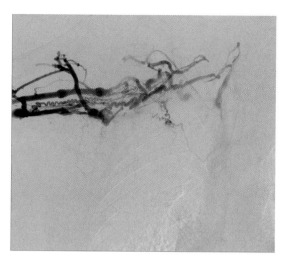

Figure 67.1

Case 67　Paget Schroetter

Figure 67.2

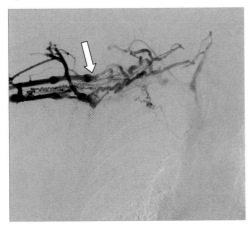

Figure 67.3

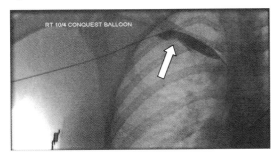

Figure 67.4

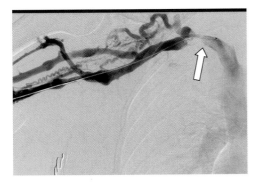

Findings

▶ Venogram demonstrates occlusion of right axillary vein (arrow, Fig. 67.2) with multiple engorged collateral veins.

▶ After subclavian vein thrombolysis, balloon venoplasty (arrow, Fig. 67.3) was performed, resulting in minimal recanalization of the subclavian vein with decrease in retrograde filling of collateral veins (Fig. 67.4). Note the waist in the balloon at the thoracic outlet (Fig. 67.4, arrow).

Teaching Points

▶ Subclavian vein effort thrombosis, or Paget Schroetter syndrome, results from compression of the subclavian vein in the thoracic outlet, which is comprised of the anterior scalene muscle, clavicle, and first rib. It may also occur in the setting of compression from a cervical rib or secondary to marked hypertrophy of the anterior scalene muscles.

▶ Symptoms include pain, swelling, and numbness of the affected arm; effort thrombosis most commonly occurs in young men who perform repetitive arm abduction, such as weight lifters or painters.

▶ The brachial plexus, subclavian vein, and artery all pass through the thoracic outlet. The majority of symptoms result from pressure on the brachial plexus, followed by the subclavian vein and artery, respectively.

Management

▶ Although contrast venography is the gold standard for diagnosis, Doppler ultrasound or magnetic resonance venography with provocative maneuvers should be obtained first to confirm the diagnosis.

▶ Thrombolysis is usually the first treatment modality to recannalize the occluded vein. This is typically followed by early surgical decompression of the thoracic outlet by resection of the cervical or first rib and anterior scale muscle. In some cases, a trial of anticoagulation prior to surgery may be considered with surgical intervention reserved for recurrence of symptoms.

▶ Catheter-directed thrombolysis should only be performed after a careful history to exclude any contraindications to thrombolytic agents. In this case, after the acute clot was traversed with a multi-sidehole catheter, alteplase was infused at a rate of 1 mg/h. Alternatively or in conjunction, mechanical thrombectomy may be considered.

▶ Stent placement should be considered only for patients who cannot tolerate surgery or who have recurrent thrombosis or stenosis after surgical decompression.

Further Reading

Thompson RW. Comprehensive management of subclavian vein effort thrombosis. *Semin Intervent Radiol.* 2012; 29(1):44–51.

History

▶ A 2-Month-Old Female with Right Neck Swelling. What Are the Treatment Options for the Lesion Shown?

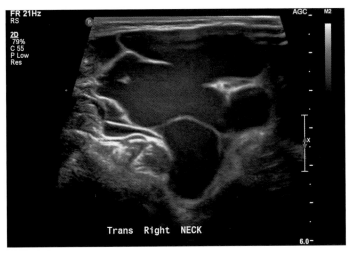

Figure 68.1

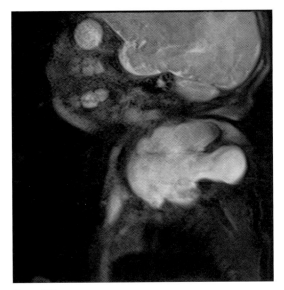

Figure 68.2

Case 68   Sclerosis of Lymphatic Malformation

Figure 68.3

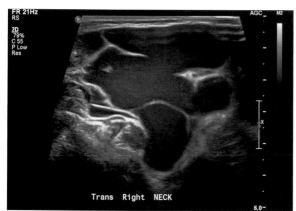

Figure 68.4

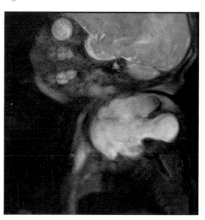

Figure 68.5

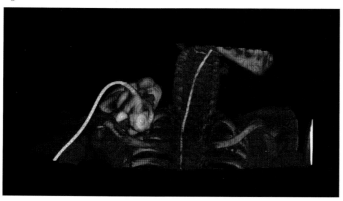

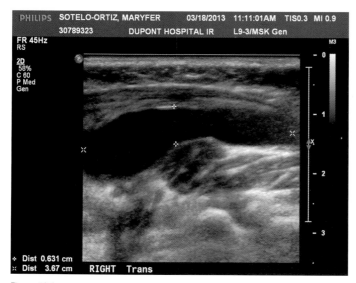

Figure 68.6

Findings

▶ Ultrasound of the right neck demonstrates multilocular thin-walled macrocysts (Fig. 68.3). No flow was seen within the cysts (not shown).

▶ T2-weighted saggital magnetic resonance image (MRI) (Fig. 68.4) shows high signal intensity consistent with fluid-filled cysts. Note macrolobulations within the lesion similar to those seen on ultrasound.

▶ A catheter was placed directly into the malformation using ultrasound guidance (not shown). Coronal computed tomography (CT) reconstruction shows the catheter within the lesion (Fig. 68.5).

▶ Follow-up ultrasound 8 weeks after sclerosis (Fig. 68.6) demonstrates significant reduction in the size of the lymphatic malformation with near-normal cosmesis.

Teaching Points

▶ The International Society of the Study of Vascular Anomalies Classification System separates vascular proliferative neoplasms from vascular malformations based on the presence or absence of endothelial proliferation.

▶ Vascular malformations are further divided into high-flow and slow-flow types. Lymphatic malformations are classified as slow-flow vascular malformations.

▶ Lymphatic malformations represent 5% of benign tumors in infancy and childhood. They occur when embryonic lymphatics fail to join central channels or secondary to congenital obstruction of lymphatic drainage.

▶ Lymphatic malformations of the neck (previously referred to as "cystic hygromas") are associated with Turner syndrome; trisomies 13, 18, 21, 22; Noonan syndrome; and exposure to teratogens.

Treatment

▶ Primary modalities used to imaging vascular malformations include ultrasound and MRI because of the lack of ionizing radiation and ability to characterize blood flow and extent of lesions.

▶ Microcystic malformations are more resistant to chemical sclerosis than macrocystic lesions and may require thermal ablation or surgical resection.

▶ Sclerosants used for lymphatic malformations include ethanol, doxycycline, and bleomycin. Doxycycline can be used effectively because it can be given in large volumes. OK-432 (Pacibinal), a combination of a low-virulence strain of Streptococcus pyogenes and benzylpenecillin, has been used with success in Japan and Europe but is not FDA approved in the United States.

▶ In this case, a pigtail catheter was placed and the lymphatic malformation treated for 3 successive days.

Further Reading

Gilony D, Schwartz M, Shpitzer T, et al. Treatment of lymphatic malformations: a more conservative approach. *J Pediatr Surg.* 2012; 47(10):1837–1842.

Lowe LH, Marchant TC, Rivard DC, et al. Vascular malformations: classification and terminology the radiologist needs to know. *Semin Roentgenol.* 2012; 47(2):106–117.

History

▶ Left Lower-Extremity Varicose Veins and Swelling

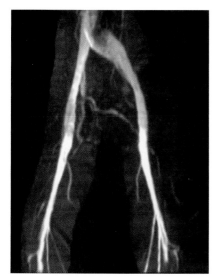

Figure 69.1

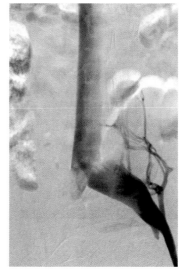

Figure 69.2

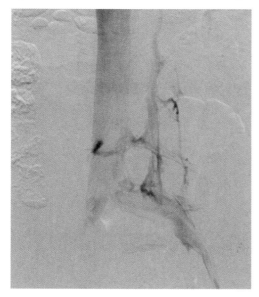

Figure 69.3

Case 69   May Thurner Syndrome

Figure 69.4

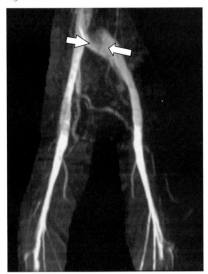

Figure 69.5

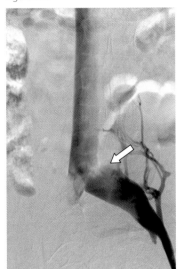

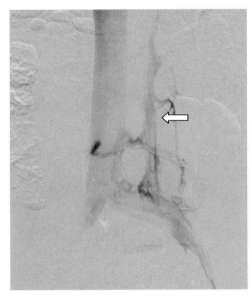

Figure 69.6

Findings

▶ Coronal magnetic resonance image (MRI) (Fig. 69.4) demonstrates compression and narrowing of the left common iliac vein at the confluence with the right. The area of narrowing conforms to the shape of the overlying right iliac artery (arrows).

▶ Narrowing of the left common iliac vein is confirmed at venography (arrow, Fig. 69.5). Collateral lumbar and hemiazygous veins are seen (arrow, Fig. 69.6). No deep venous thrombosis was seen (not shown).

Teaching Points

▶ May Thurner syndrome, or iliac vein compression syndrome, results from compression of the left common iliac vein between the right common iliac artery and spine at the level of the sacral promontory.

▶ May Thurner accounts for <4% of lower-extremity deep venous thrombosis. It is most common in young to middle-age females and should be considered in the setting of chronic unilateral left leg swelling or varicosities.

▶ Patients usually present with acute-onset left leg swelling and pain.

▶ The combination of mechanical compression and pulsatile vibrations from the right common iliac artery causes chronic microtrauma, leading to endothelial injury.

Treatment

▶ Treatment is dependent on symptomatology. Conservative treatment includes use of compression stockings and elevation of the leg when possible.

▶ In the presence of deep venous thrombosis, endovascular pharmacological and/or mechanical thrombolysis with venous stent placement can be considered. Early thrombolysis is critical in preventing postthrombotic syndrome, which can include pain, paresthesias, swelling, varicose veins, skin discoloration, and ulcer.

▶ When stent placement is indicated, self-expanding stents are used because, unlike balloon expandable stents, they are not subject to the deformity due to extrinsic compression.

▶ Following stent placement, anticoagulation and compression stockings are recommended to prevent recurrence.

Further Reading

Butros SR, Liu R, Oliveira GR, et al. Venous compression syndromes: clinical features, imaging findings and management. *Br J Radiol*. 2013; 86(1030):20130284.

History

▶ A 45-Year-Old Female Status Post Recent Resection of Craniopharyngioma with Postoperative Pulmonary Embolism, Referred for Inferior Vena Cava Filter Placement

Figures 70.1 and 70.2 are of two different patients. What is the difference?

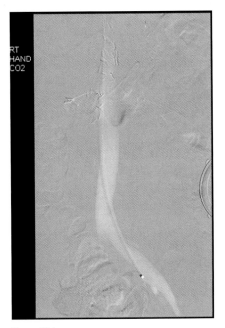

Figure 70.1

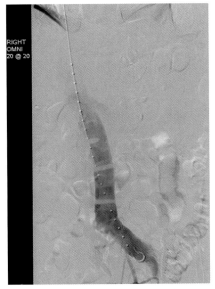

Figure 70.2

Case 70 Inferior Vena Cava Filter Placement

Figure 70.1

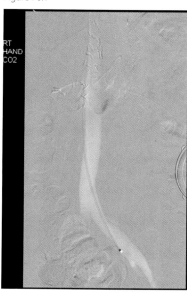

Figure 70.2

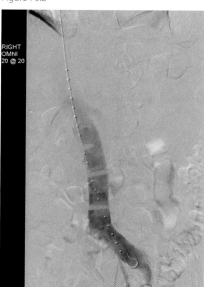

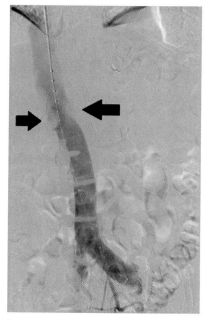

Figure 70.3

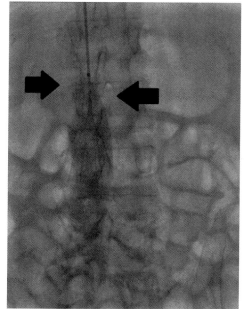

Figure 70.4

Findings

▶ Figure 70.1 depicts an inferior venacavagram performed with the catheter tip within the left common iliac vein. Carbon dioxide gas is used as the contrast agent because the patient has an anaphylactic reaction to iodinated contrast.

▶ Figure 70.2 demonstrates a typical inferior venocavagram performed with iodinated contrast.

- An inferior venocavagram is performed to identify intraluminal thrombus, the size of the cava, duplication anomalies, and the level of the renal veins as demonstrated by the inflow defect representing non-contrast-enhanced blood return from the renal veins into the column of the opacified vena cava (Fig. 70.3, black arrows).
- The inferior vena caval filter is placed in an infrarenal location (Fig. 70.4). The black arrows demonstrate the renal inflow on the postdeployment cavagram.

Teaching Points

- Carbon dioxide can be used as a contrast agent in the setting of iodinated contrast allergies or renal failure.
- Currently accepted indications for IVC Filter placement in patients with documented venous thromboembolism (VTE) include patients with the following:
  - Contraindication to anticoagulation or inability to maintain adequate anticoagulation
  - Documented progression or recurrence of VTE while on anticoagulation
  - Complications from anticoagulation
  - Massive pulmonary embolism requiring thrombolysis or surgical thrombectomy
- With increased used of retrievable filters, indications for use continue to expand which can include the following:
  - Prophylaxis in patients at risk for VTE who may be bedbound for a prolonged period due to trauma or surgery
  - Patients with large clot burdens such as iliocaval deep vein thrombosis or thrombus in the inferior vena cava
- The current line of filters can be placed in inferior vena cavae measuring up to 28 mm.
- If a megacava is identified, a Bird's Nest permanent filter can be placed in cava measuring between 28 and 40 mm. Bilateral iliac filters should be placed in cavae measuring greater than 40 mm.
- IVC filters should be placed just below the renal inflows.

Management

- With the increased use of retrievable filters, patients should be educated about early retrieval of these filters once risk of VTE returns to normal.
- Internal jugular approach is preferred when possible for ease of catheterizing the left iliac vein to exclude duplication anomaly, the ability to capture and move unexpected thrombosis caudally to allow for infrarenal filter position, and for patient comfort in recovering in a seated rather than supine position.

Further Reading

Harvey JJ, Hopkins J, McCafferty IJ, et al. Inferior vena caval filters: what radiologists need to know. *Clin Radiol*. 2013; 68(7):721–732.

History

▶ Intractable Abdominal Pain Status Post Inferior Vena Cava Filter Placement

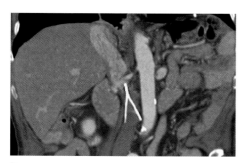

Figure 71.1

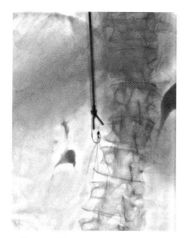

Figure 71.2

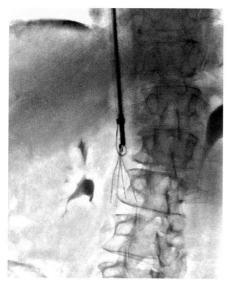

Figure 71.3

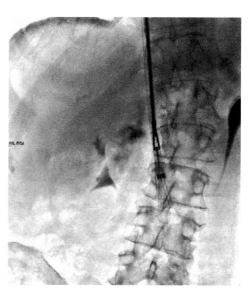

Figure 71.4

Case 71   Inferior Vena Cava Filter Removal

Figure 71.5

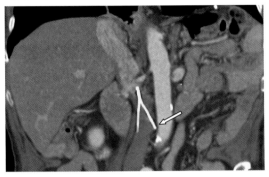

Figure 71.6

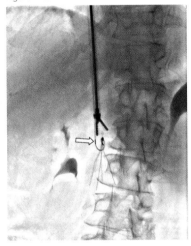

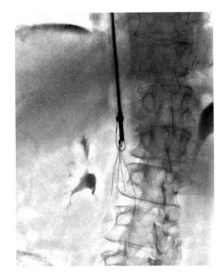

Figure 71.7

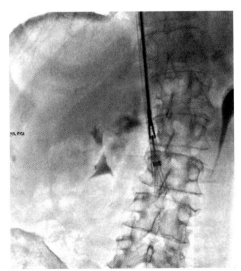

Figure 71.8

Findings

▶ Coronal computed tomography (CT) reconstruction shows an inferior vena cava (IVC) filter in the infrarenal IVC (Fig. 71.5). The IVC is tortous, and relative to the axis of the vessel, the filter is mildly tilted. The medial leg of the filter appears to be protruding through the wall of the vessel (arrow).

▶ A tip-deflecting wire (Fig. 71.6, arrow) is seen under the hook at the neck of the filter. This was used to free the filter from its position against the wall of the cava, making the hook accessible for capture. After a loop snare failed to snare the hook, an alligator forceps was used (71.6 arrow and 71.7). Once the forceps grasped the hook, the sheath was advanced over the filter which was removed without further difficulty (Fig. 71.8).

Teaching Points

▶ Truly temporary filters must be removed and are rarely, if ever, used; almost all filters currently being placed are retrievable filters approved for permanent implantation, for example, the Gunther Tulip ©, Option ©, and Trapese ©.

▶ The incidence of deep vein thrombosis is increased by the presence of a filter, and the risk increases over time. Removal of IVC filters, when appropriate, is performed to reduce the sequela of venous incompetence and caval thrombosis.

▶ Early removal increases likelihood of success. Within 3 months, over 90% can be successfully removed, decreasing to under half at 1 year.

▶ Filters can be difficult to remove if the hook is embedded in the wall or becomes unformed during the attempt. In such cases, a tip-deflecting wire or balloon displacement can be used to reposition the hook into the lumen of the IVC. Alternatively, a "sling" technique can be used in which a reverse-curve catheter is advanced distal to the filter and a wire advanced out of the catheter (extending cranial to the filter) can be snared, allowing the filter to be pulled into the guiding sheath and removed.

▶ IVC perforation is defined as any part, usually a leg, of the filter extending >3 mm beyond the wall of the IVC. Perforation can result in pain or injury to adjacent structures.

▶ There are currently no prospective trials comparing efficacy and complications of different filter designs.

Management

▶ Prior to removing a filter, a cavogram should be performed to assess for trapped thrombus. When present, clot that occupies >25% of the volume of the filter precludes removal in most cases.

▶ The most common causes of failed retrieval is endothelization of the legs in the wall of the cava.

Further Reading

Iliescu B, Haskal ZJ. Adanced techniques for removal of retrievable inferior vena cava filters. *Cardiovasc Intervent Radiol.* 2012; 35(4):741–750.

PREPIC (Prevention du Risque d'Embolie Pulmonaire par Interrruption Cave) Study Group. Eight year follow up of patients with permanent vena cava filters in the prevention of pulmonary embolism: the PREPIC randomized study. *Circulation* 2005; 112:416–422.

History

▶ A 60-Year-Old Female with Chronic Indwelling Permanent Inferior Vena Cava Filter Placed 6 Years Prior Presents with Several-Month History of Chronic Bilateral Leg Swelling with 1 Week of Acute Worsening

Based on findings seen on Figures 72.1–72.5, is there a potential treatment for this patient?

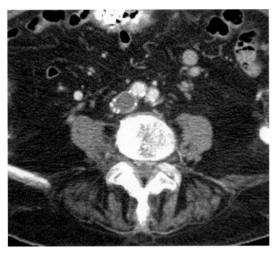

Figure 72.1

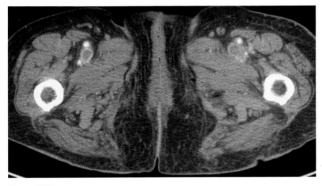

Figure 72.2

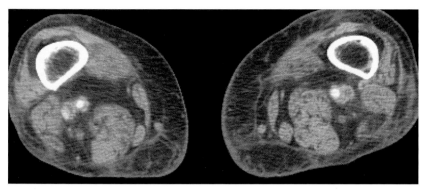

Figure 72.3

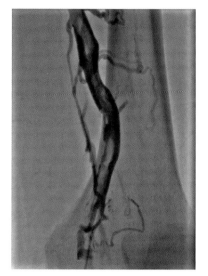

Figure 72.4

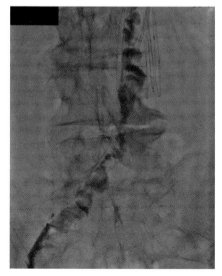

Figure 72.5

Case 72   Inferior Vena Cava Stent

Acute on chronic thrombosis of the venous system below a permanent inferior vena cava (IVC) filter extending to the above-knee popliteal veins bilaterally. This patient could potentially undergo bilateral venous lysis.

Figure 72.3

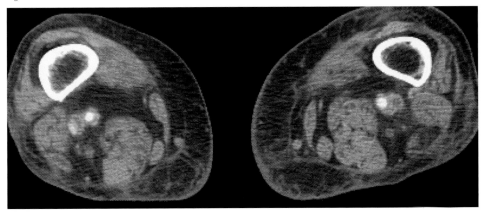

Figure 72.6

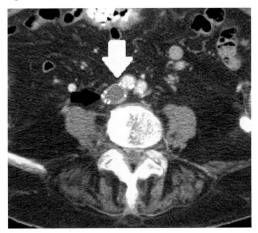

Figure 72.7

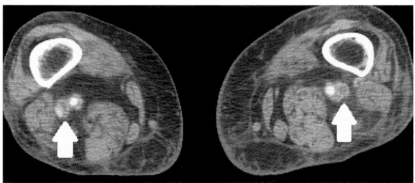

Figure 72.8

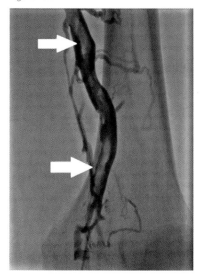

Figure 72.9

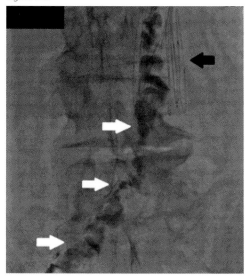

Figure 72.10

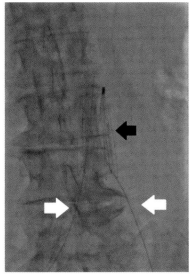

Figure 72.11   Figure 72.12

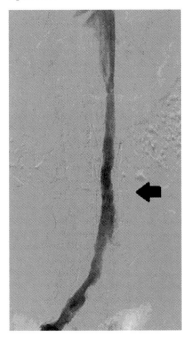

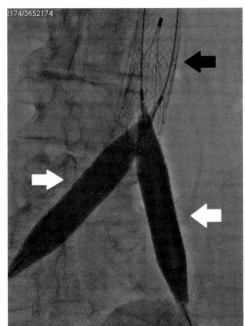

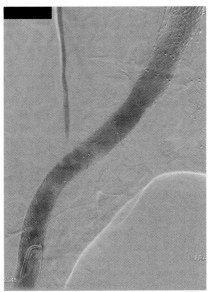

Figure 72.13

Findings

▶ Contrast-enhanced computed tomography (CT) (Figs. 72.6, 72.3, and 72.7) demonstrates complete occlusion with extensive thrombus extending from the infrarenal IVC filter (Fig. 72.6 arrow) to the popliteal veins bilaterally (Fig. 72.7, arrows).

▶ Selective venograms from the right lower extremity (Figs. 72.8 and 72.9) demonstrate filling defects within the femoral vein (arrows, Fig. 72.8) representing acute clot, with irregularity of the right common iliac vein (white arrows, Fig. 72.9) representing chronic changes extending to a permanent IVC filter (black arrow, Fig. 72.9).

▶ Bilateral lysis catheters (white arrows, Fig. 72.10) extending from just above the IVC filter (black arrow, Fig. 72.10) to the popliteal veins were left with a 24-hour alteplase infusion at a total rate of 1.0 mg/hr.

- After 24 hours of alteplase infusion, venogram (Fig. 72.11) shows improved flow through the filter (black arrow).
- Decision was made to stent across the IVC filter (black arrow, Fig. 72.12) with re-creation of the iliac vein confluence (white arrows, Fig. 72.12).
- After lysis and stent placement, a venogram (Fig. 72.13) depicts a widely patent right common iliac vein and IVC.

Teaching Points

- Unlike iliofemoral deep vein thrombosis (see Case 73), there are no established indications for recanalization of a chronically occluded IVC.
- Prior to intervention, physical examination and imaging are critical to evaluate the extent of clot burden and to identify involvement of hepatic or renal vein inflows, which may affect stent landing sites.
- Chronically imbedded filters can be stented open with a high-radial-force, self-expanding stent such as a Wallstent ©.
- Self-expanding stents are used because of their ability to re-expand when an external force is removed. Balloon expandable stents are prone to crush when confronted with external forces.

Management

- Stenting is performed with ACT 250–300 seconds.
- After IVC recanalization and stent placement, anticoagulation is suggested for 2–3 months.
- Follow up with patient at 3, 6, and 12 months and annually after procedure with ultrasound. Repeat venogram is performed in the setting of increased symptoms or if the ultrasound identifies areas of abnormality.

Further Reading

Bjarnason H. Tips and tricks for stenting the inferior vena cava. *Semin Vasc Surg.* 2013; 26:29–34.
Neglen P, Oglesbee M, Olivier J, et al. Stenting of chronically obstructed inferior vena cava filters. *J Vasc Surg.* 2011;54:153–161.

History

▶ A 74-Year-Old Male with History of Lymphoma with Acute Lower-Extremity Swelling

A computed tomography (CT) is shown in Figures 73.1 and 73.2. Describe the procedure in Figures 73.3 and 73.4. Figure 73.5 represents the follow-up after the procedure. What else can be done?

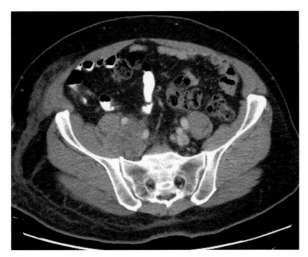

Figure 73.1

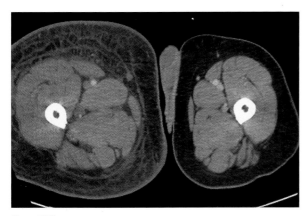

Figure 73.2

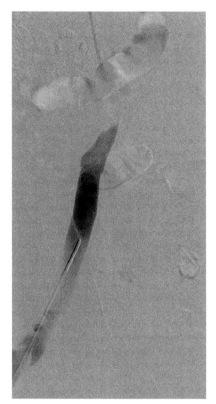

Figure 73.3

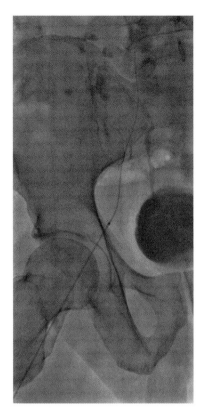

Figure 73.4

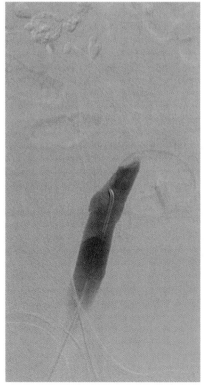

Figure 73.5

Case 73 Lower-Extremity Lysis

Acute on chronic right lower-extremity deep vein thrombosis (DVT) with external compression from an enlarged lymph node. A stent was subsequently deployed.

Figure 73.2

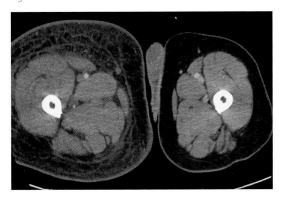

Figure 73.6

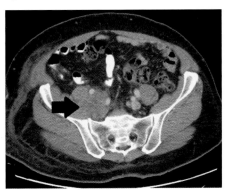

Figure 73.7

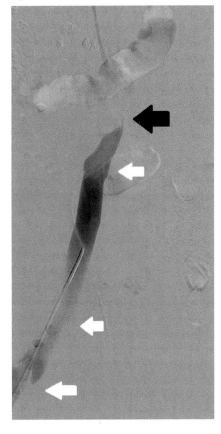

Figure 73.8

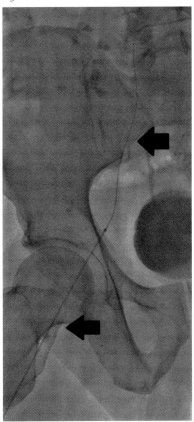

Figure 73.9

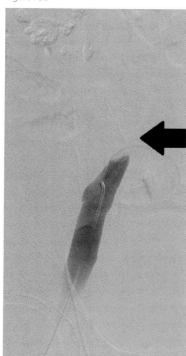

Figure 73.10

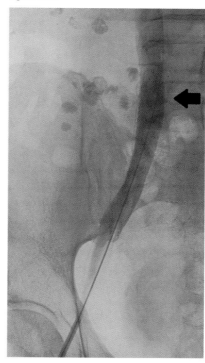

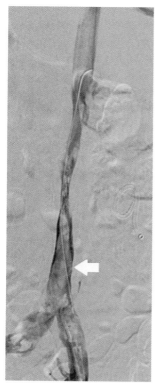

Figure 73.11

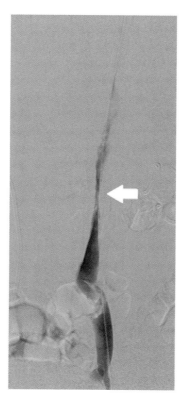

Figure 73.12

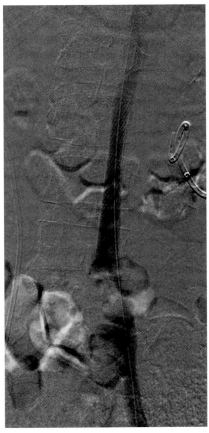

Figure 73.13

Findings

► Figures 73.6 and 73.2 demonstrate asymmetric soft tissue edema in the right lower extremity with enlarged lymph nodes compressing and obliterating the right common iliac vein (black arrow).
► Figure 73.7 demonstrates a venogram performed in the right common iliac vein with significant stenosis of the vein secondary to external compression (black arrow) with multiple filling defects likely representing acute thrombus (white arrows).
► Figure 73.8 show a lysis catheter across the area of stenosis and across all the documented thrombus (black arrows).
► Figure 73.9 show persistent stenosis (black arrow) despite clot lysis after overnight alteplase drip.
► Figure 73.10 demonstrates interval placement of a self-expanding stent across the stenosis with good angiographic result (black arrow).
► Figure 73.11–73.13 is a companion case demonstrating acute clot in the inferior vena cava (IVC) extending to the common iliac veins bilaterally (filling defects in Figure 73.11, white arrow). The patient underwent subsequent catheter-directed thrombolysis with residual IVC stenosis (Fig. 73.12, white arrow) necessitating stent placement (Fig. 73.13).

Teaching Points

An American Heart Association (AHA) statement regarding management of DVT suggests the following:

► With regard to iliofemoral deep venous thrombosis (IFDVT) where clot burden includes partial or complete thrombosis of the iliac vein or the common femoral vein, with or without proximal or distal extension, initial treatment should include therapeutic doses of unfractionated heparin, low molecular weight heparin (LMWH), or fondaparinux.

- Long-term anticoagulation includes use of warfarin with target International Normalized Ratio (INR) of 2.0–3.0 for at least 3 months for first episode of IFDVT with a major reversible risk factor or at least 6 months for recurrent or unprovoked IFDVT and considered for lifelong anticoagulation.
- Cancer patients with IFDVT should receive LMWH for at least 3–6 months or for as long as cancer therapy is ongoing.
- Catheter-directed or pharmacomechanical catheter-directed thrombolysis:
  - Should be performed for patients with limb-threatening compromise.
  - Is reasonable for patients with rapidly extending IFDVT.
  - Is reasonable as first-line therapy to prevent postthrombotic syndrome.
- Regarding venoplasty or stent placement:
  - Stent placement after catheter-directed or pharmacomechanical catheter-directed thrombolysis for obstructive lesions in the iliac vein is reasonable.
  - For isolated femoral vein obstructive lesions, a trial of venoplasty without stenting is reasonable.
  - Placement of iliac stents to reduce symptoms of postthrombotic syndrome and to heal nonhealing ulcers is reasonable.

Management

- After venous stenting, long-term anticoagulation recommendations for IFDVT apply.
- Use of antiplatelet drugs in addition to anticoagulation may be considered for those perceived to be at high risk.

Further Reading

Jaff MR, McMurtry S, Aracher SL, et al. Management of massive and submassive pulmonary embolism, illiofemoral deep venous thrombosis, and chronic thromboembolic pulmonary hypertension. *Circulation*. 2011; 123:1788–1830.

History

▶ A 57-Year-Old Female with History of Metastatic Ovarian Cancer Presents with Acute Shortness of Breath

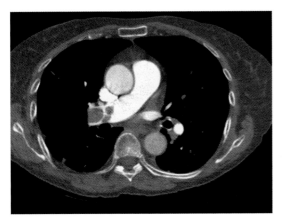

Figure 74.1

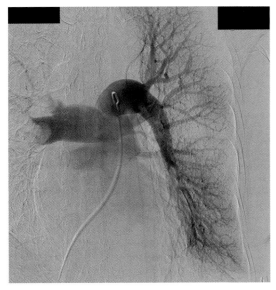

Figure 74.2

Case 74   Acute Pulmonary Embolism

Figure 74.3

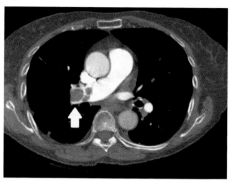

Figure 74.4

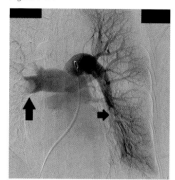

Figure 74.5

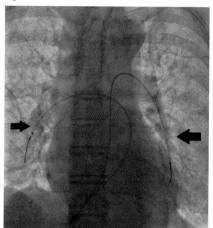

Figure 74.6

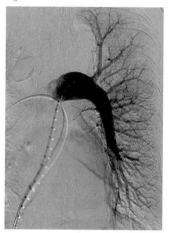

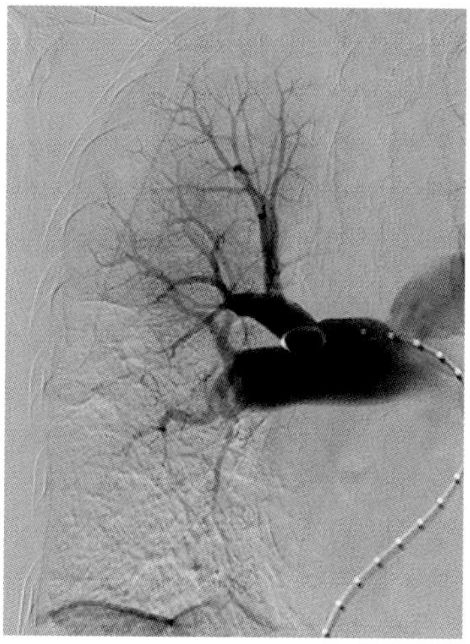

Figure 74.7

Figure 74.8

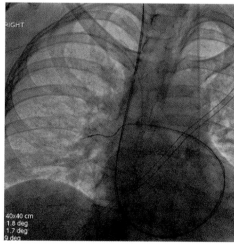

Findings

▶ A large pulmonary embolism within the right main pulmonary artery (Fig. 74.3, white arrow)

▶ Left main pulmonary arteriogram shows filling defects within the left lower lobe segmental pulmonary artery (small black arrow, Fig. 74.4) and a large embolism within the right main pulmonary artery (large black arrow, Fig. 74.4).

▶ Bilateral infusion catheters were placed across the clot (black arrows, Fig. 74.5) and alteplase was infused over 24 hours.

▶ Postlysis angiograms show resolution of the clot within the left lower lobe segmental branch (Fig. 74.6) and marked improvement in the right main filling defect (Fig. 74.7).

▶ Figure 74.8 shows a rotation thrombectomy system being used in a different patient with extensive right pulmonary artery clot burden.

Teaching Points

▶ Multiple potential therapies exist for treatment of acute pulmonary embolism ranging from systemic anticoagulation for the stable patient to catheter-directed thrombolysis/mechanical thrombectomy or surgical thrombectomy for the unstable patient with massive pulmonary emboli.

▶ Endovascular therapies include chemical thrombolysis (pulse or overnight) and mechanical thrombolysis such as disruption of clot with a pigtail catheter and rotational devices like the Cleaner (Rex Medical, Conshohocken, PA), shown in Figure 74.8.

▶ Thorough thrombolysis in the setting of submassive pulmonary embolism has the potential of reducing the development of chronic hypertension due to chronic pulmonary embolism.

Management

An American Heart Association (AHA) statement regarding management of acute pulmonary embolism suggests the following:

▶ Assuming no contraindications, therapeutic systemic anticoagulation should be started for confirmed pulmonary embolism. Patients with clinically intermediate or high probability for pulmonary embolism should be started on empiric anticoagulation during the workup.

▶ Catheter-based therapy can be considered in patients with massive pulmonary embolism with contraindications to fibrinolysis and in patients who remain unstable after receiving fibrinolysis.

▶ Catheter-based therapy may be considered in patients with submassive acute pulmonary embolism judged to have clinical evidence of adverse prognosis (new hemodynamic instability, worsening respiratory failure, severe right ventricular dysfunction, or major myocardial necrosis).

▶ Catheter-based therapies are not recommended for patients with low-risk pulmonary embolism or submassive acute pulmonary embolism with minor right ventricular dysfunction, minor myocardial necrosis, and no clinical worsening.

Further Reading

Jaff MR, McMurtry S, Aracher SL, et al. Management of massive and submassive pulmonary embolism, illiofemoral deep venous thrombosis, and chronic thromboembolic pulmonary hypertension. *Circulation.* 2011; 123:1788–1830.

Kuo, WT, Gould MK, Louie JD, et al. Catheter-directed therapy for the treatment of massive pulmonary embolism: systematic review and meta-analysis of modern techniques. *J Vasc Interv Radiol.* 2009; 20:1431–1440.

History

▶ A 50-Year-Old Male with Intracranial Metastasis Presents with Acute Lower-Extremity Deep Vein Thrombosis in Need of an Inferior Vena Cava Filter

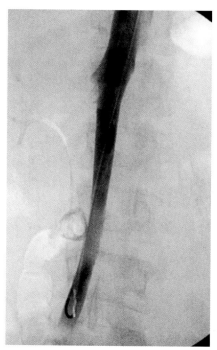

Figure 75.1

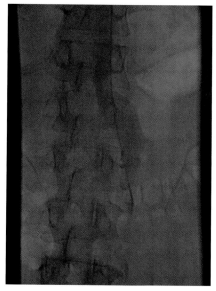

Figure 75.2

Case 75 Duplicated Inferior Vena Cava

Figure 75.3

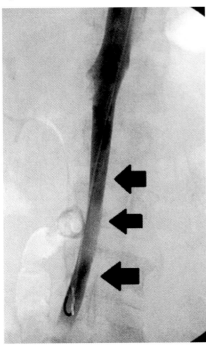

Figure 75.4

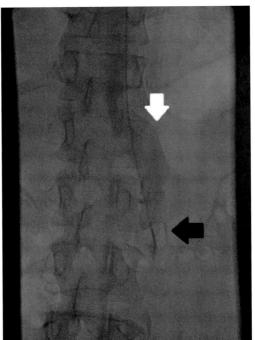

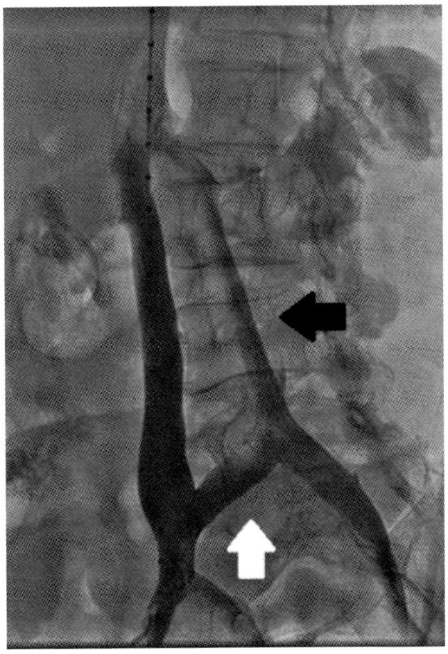

Figure 75.5

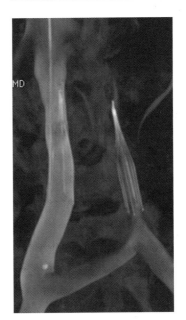

Figure 75.6

Findings

▶ Inferior venacavagram (Fig. 75.3) performed from an internal jugular approach shows catheter tip position in the right common iliac vein. The inferior vena cava (IVC) is relatively narrow, and at the expected confluence of iliac veins the IVC is very smooth; there is no obvious inflow from the left common iliac vein (black arrows).

▶ The left renal vein was subsequently catheterized (Fig. 75.4), confirming the diagnosis of a duplicated IVC (black arrow), which drains into the left renal vein (white arrow).

▶ Figure 75.5 is an inferior venacavagram from a different patient with a duplicated IVC (black arrow), demonstrating communication between the two below the renal veins (white arrow).

▶ Conebeam computed tomography (CT) venogram of the same patient in Figure 75.5 after placement of two retrievable filters, one in each IVC (Fig. 75.6).

Teaching Points

▶ Preplacement inferior venacavagrams are performed to evaluate for the presence of intraluminal thrombus, aberrant anatomy, the size of the cava, and the location of the renal vein inflow.

▶ To confirm that there are not anatomic anomalies of the IVC, the catheter tip should be placed in the left common iliac vein.

▶ Duplication of the IVC occurs in 0.2%–3% of the population.

▶ Filtration needs to include both cavae. Placement of a filter in each cava is preferred, but if not technically feasible, a single IVC filter can be placed in a suprarenal position.

▶ Duplication of the IVC can be varied in appearance with no communication between the two cavae or communication below the renal veins, as demonstrated in Figures 75.3 and 75.4.

▶ Other common caval anomalies and suggested filter locations:
  ▪ Circumaortic left renal vein—place filter below the orifice of the retrocaval component.
  ▪ Retroaortic left renal vein—place filter below orifice of the left renal vein if space allows; otherwise consider bilateral common iliac vein filters or suprarenal filter.

Management

▶ As with single retrievable filters, patients and referring physicians should be educated on the optimal time interval for retrieval once risk of venous thromboembolic disease returns to normal.

Further Reading

Bass EJ, Redwine MD, Kramer LA, et al. Spectrum of congenital anomalies of the inferior vena cava: cross-sectional imaging findings. *Radiographics*. 2000; 20:639–652.

History

▶ Figures 76.1 and 76.2 demonstrate a patient who presents to the emergency department with acute back pain. Discuss important findings to identify on the computed tomography (CT). Figures 76.3–76.5 show a different patient with more acute symptoms requiring endovascular and subsequent surgical therapy. What is being done?

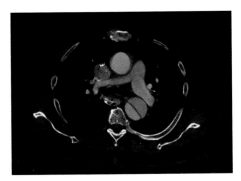

Figure 76.1

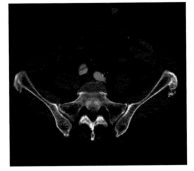

Figure 76.2

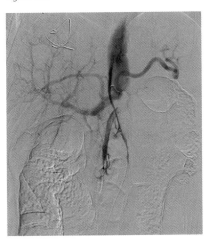

Figure 76.3

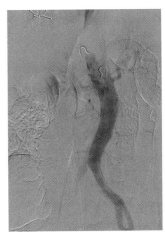

Figure 76.4

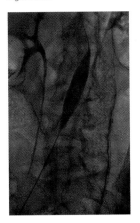

Figure 76.5

Case 76 Type B Aortic Dissection and Fenestration

Figure 76.6

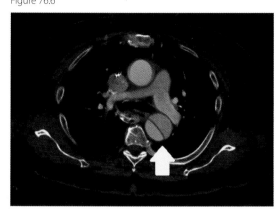

Figure 76.7

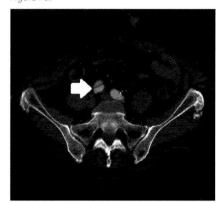

Figure 76.8

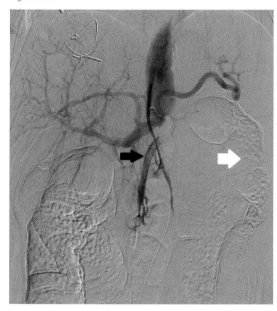

Figure 76.9

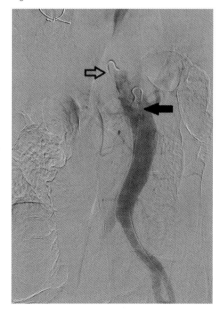

Figure 76.10

Figure 76.11

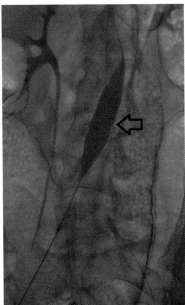

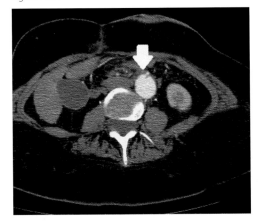

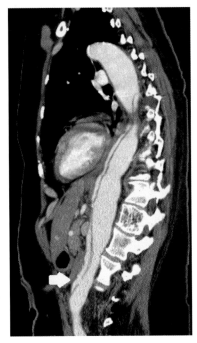

Figure 76.12

Findings

▶ Figures 76.6 and 76.7, show the CT scan from the emergency department presentation showing a type B aortic dissection (arrow) extending to right left common iliac artery.

▶ In a different patient with right lower-extremity symptoms with no definite abdominal symptoms, aortic fenestration was performed. Figure 76.8 shows a catheter in the false lumen that supplies the celiac system and superior mesenteric artery (SMA). Unfortunately, at this point, thrombus was noted in the SMA (black arrow) and pneumatosis was seen on fluoroscopic images (white arrow). On discussion with the surgeon, given the right lower-extremity symptoms, fenestration was performed with subsequent abdominal exploration.

► Figure 76.9 show flush catheters in both true and false lumens from bilateral common femoral arterial access (arrows).

► Figure 76.10 shows a balloon fenestration after access was achieved between the two lumens.

► Figures 76.11 and 76.12 show a CT angiogram performed 6 months after treatment showing flow in both true and false lumen with fenestration seen (arrow). Note the patient has undergone total colectomy for ischemic colitis related to the initial presentation.

Teaching Points

► Stanford type A dissections originate in the ascending aorta and are managed surgically.

► Stanford type B dissections originate in the descending aorta and are generally managed medically with strict blood pressure control.

► Type A dissections that are surgically treated or type B dissections may go on to develop visceral vascular compromise such as mesenteric, renal, or peripheral ischemia, which is refractory to medical management. This group may require emergent endovascular or open surgical fenestration to create a communication between the false and true lumens to restore flow to the affected organ.

► The aim of fenestration is to try and equalize the pressure gradient between the false and true lumens to allow visceral vessel reperfusion.

► General Technique
  - Access is obtained to the true and false lumens. Pressure gradients are obtained. If there is no significant gradient, fenestration is unlikely to be helpful.
  - When fenestration is decided upon, a "target" is placed in the false lumen (snare or pigtail/Sos catheter). A hollow metal needle is advanced via a sheath from the true lumen to the area to be fenestrated.
  - Most common needle systems include needles from a transjugular liver biopsy kit. The needle is advanced into the "target" in the false lumen. Entry into the false lumen is confirmed via angiography or intravascular ultrasound (IVUS).
  - The fenestration is dilated to 15 mm over a stiff wire. Pressures are remeasured and angiograms performed, looking for visceral vessel reperfusion.
  - Once fenestration is performed, stents can be placed in the true lumen of the hemodynamically significant or symptomatic branch vessel lesions. Priority is usually given to the superior mesenteric artery over the celiac artery, followed by one kidney.

Management

► There is little consensus on appropriate follow-up for these patients as very few sites have extensive experience. It is clear that lifelong imaging surveillance is prudent.

Further Reading

Hartnell GG, Gates J. Aortic fenestration: a why, when and how-to guide. *Radiographics*. 2005; 25:175–189.

History

▶ An 84-Year-Old Male with History of Hypertension and Diabetes Status post Endovascular Aneurysm Repair of a 6 cm Infrarenal Abdominal Aortic Aneurysm Three Years Ago

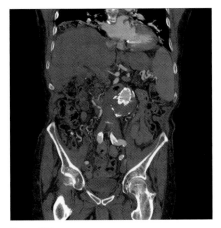

Figure 77.1

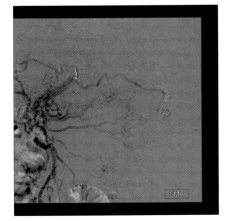

Figure 77.2

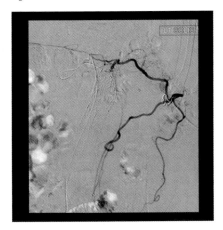

Figure 77.3

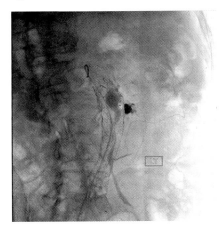

Figure 77.4

Case 77   Endoleak

Figure 77.5

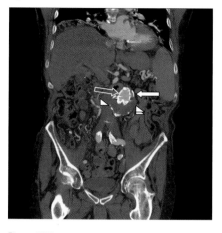

Figure 77.6

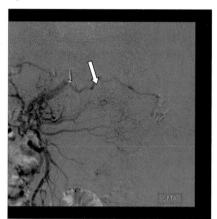

Figure 77.7

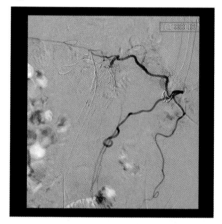

Figure 77.8

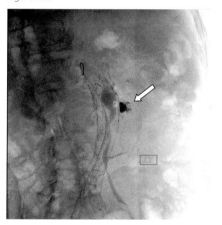

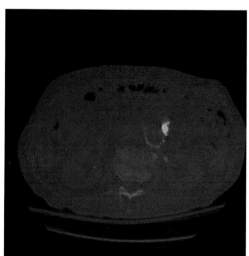

Figure 77.9

Findings

▶ Coronal reformat of contrast-enhanced computed tomography (CT) (Fig. 77.5) shows an abdominal aortic aneurysm (arrowheads) with an indwelling aortic stent graft (hollow arrow.) Contrast is seen in the excluded aneurysm adjacent to an enhancing vessel (arrow).

▶ Superior mesenteric angiogram (Figs. 77.6 and 77.7) shows communication between the superior mesenteric artery and the left colic artery (a branch of the inferior mesenteric artery) via the arc of Riolan.

▶ A distal branch of the left colic artery supplying the endoleak was catheterized via the superior mesenteric artery and embolized with Onyx (Fig. 77.8, arrow). Noncontrast CT image after endoleak embolization shows retention of Onyx in the aneurysm sac (Fig. 77.9).

Teaching Points

▶ Endoleak refers to continued pressurization and enlargement of the aneurysm sac despite exclusion by the aortic endograft.

▶ Detection of endoleaks are important because persistent filling of the aneurysm sac results in increased pressure and/or enlargement of the sac, predisposing to rupture.

▶ Endoleaks have been classified based on their source by a consensus panel of vascular surgeons and interventional radiologists:

    Type I endoleaks occur at attachment sites of the stent graft.

    Type II refers to reperfusion of the sac from aortic branches. These are the most common type of endoleak. The case shown is a typical example of a type II endoleak caused by a branch of the left colic artery.

    Type III is a failure of the graft itself, either the metallic lattice or fabric lining.

    Type IV is caused by increased porosity of the fabric. These are very rare in clinical practice.

    Type V refers to the situation in which the aneurysm sac enlarges but no endoleak can be found.

Management

▶ Short-interval follow up with a contrast-enhanced study (CT, US, MRI) should be obtained after endovascular repair to evaluate for primary endoleak (i.e., within 30 days of placement) and to evaluate for shrinkage of the aneurysm sac. Follow-up thereafter is institution dependent, usually at least annually.

▶ The Society for Vascular Surgery guidelines addressing post-EVAR surveillance recommend triple-phase CT angiogram at 30 days and 12 months post endovascular aneurysm repair (EVAR). If an endoleak or aneurysm sac growth is seen on the 30-day CT angiogram, 6-month follow-up CT angiogram is recommended. If there is no endoleak, device abnormality, or aneurysm sac enlargement at 30 days and 12 months, surveillance with annual color duplex ultrasound in an accredited noninvasive vascular laboratory is an accepted alternative to CT angiogram.

▶ Treatment of a type II endoleak is indicated if it is associated with enlargement of the aneurysm sac. The most common culprits include branches of the lumbar, inferior mesenteric, or middle sacral artery. Ongoing surveillance after treatment of a type II endoleak is important, as up to 20% will require a second treatment.

▶ Options to treat type II endoleaks include the transarterial approach (as shown) and direct puncture of the sac. Embolic agents used include thrombin, NBCA, and Onyx. Transarterially, coils may also be considered.

▶ Case courtesy of George G Vatakencherry MD, Kaiser Permanente Medical Group.

Further Reading

Endoleaks: Classification, diagnosis and treatment. In: Mauro MA, Murphy KPJ, Thomson KR, Venbrux AC, Morgan RA, eds. *Image Guided Interventions*. Philadelphia, PA: Elsevier Saunders; 2014:334–347.

Chaikof EL, Brewster DC, Dalman RL, et al. SVS practice guidelines for the care of patients with an abdominal aortic aneurysm: executive summary. *J Vasc Surg*. 2009; 50:880–896.

Sarac TP, Gibbons C, Vargas L, et al. Long-term follow-up of type II endoleak embolization reveals the need for close surveillance. *J Vasc Surg*. 2012; 55:33–40.

History

▶ A 25-Year-Old Male Brought in by Ambulance for Gunshot Wound to Face

Figures 78.1–78.4 show the initial computed tomography (CT) scan and arteriogram. What are the treatment options?

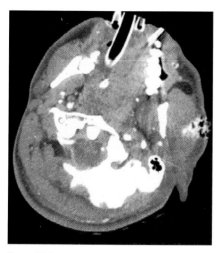

Figure 78.1

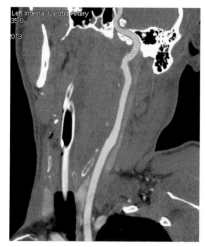

Figure 78.2

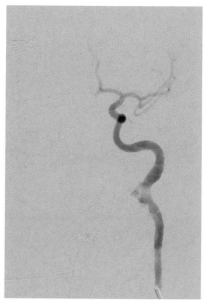

Figure 78.3

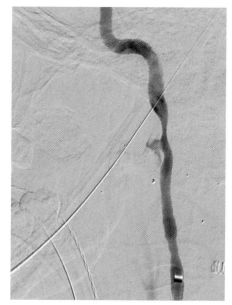

Figure 78.4

Case 78 Traumatic Pseudoaneurysm of the Carotid Artery

Carotid stenting with coil embolization of the pseudoaneurysm sac was performed.

Figure 78.5

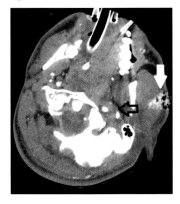

Figure 78.6

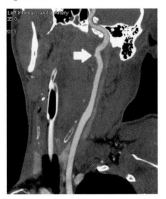

Figure 78.7

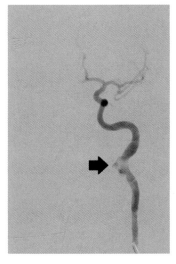

Figure 78.8

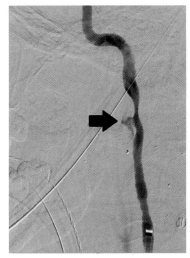

Figure 78.9

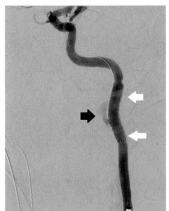

Figure 78.10

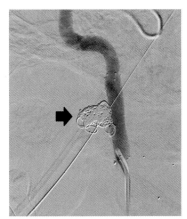

Findings

▶ Axial contrast CT demonstrates air and soft tissue swelling from the bullet entry (white arrow, Fig. 78.5). There is asymmetric soft tissue swelling of the left parapharyngeal space (black arrow, Fig. 78.5) with irregularity of the distal left internal carotid artery, better appreciated in reconstructed views (white arrow, Fig. 78.6).

▶ Frontal and lateral arteriograms (Figs. 78.7 and 78.8) of the left internal carotid artery show irregularity of the distal left internal carotid artery with contrast extravasation into a pseudoaneurysm sac.

▶ A stent was placed across the area of injury (white arrow). Initial postdeployment images show leak of contrast out the stent interstices into the pseudoaneurysm sac. Repeat angiogram after a short delayed shows this leak to persist (black arrow, Fig. 78.9).

▶ Secondary to the persistent leak, coil embolization of the sac was performed through the stent intersticces (black arrow, Fig. 78.10) with good angiographic result.

Teaching Points

▶ Pseudoaneurysms are typically saccular outpouchings that do not involve all three layers of the arterial wall (as opposed to true aneurysms).

▶ CT angiogram can underestimate the injury. Angiography should be performed if there is a high index of suspicion of vascular injury.

▶ Repair can be performed with endovascular techniques versus open repair. Open repair includes clipping, resection with primary end-to-end anastomosis or graft, exclusion and bypass, or carotid ligation.

▶ Interventional techniques to treat traumatic vessel injury or pseudoaneurysm include embolization of the vessel distal and proximal to the site of injury and covered stent placement. Covered stent placement, when feasible, is preferred because it preserves vessel patency.

▶ More typically, common carotid artery stents are placed for the treatment of carotid artery stenosis. In symptomatic patients (transient ischemic attack, amaurosis fugax, or other cerebrovascular event) the threshold for stent placement in angiographic stenoses is greater than 50%, whereas in asymptomatic patients it is greater than 70%.

Management

▶ Endovascular management was utilized here secondary to a difficult neck dissection and high carotid injury.

▶ Endovascular options include exclusion with a stent graft or stenting with coil embolization of the sac through the interstices, performed here.

▶ Stent size should be 10%–20% larger than the diameter of the vessel proximal to the injured (or in the case of atherosclerotic disease, stenotic) site.

▶ Anticoagulation following stent placement is important to prevent stent occlusion. In the setting of trauma, as in this case, it may need to be delayed. Anticoagulation following arterial stent placement typically includes antiplatelet agents such as aspirin and clopidogrel.

Further Reading

Brott TG, Hobson RW, Howard G et al. Stenting versus endarterectomy for treatment of carotid-artery stenosis. *N Engl J Med.* 2010; 313:11–23.

Garg K, Rockman CB, Lee V, et al. Presentation and management of carotid artery aneurysms and pseudoaneurysms. *J Vasc Surg.* 2012; 55(6):1618–1622.

History

▶ A 50-Year-Old Female in High-Speed Motor Vehicle Collision

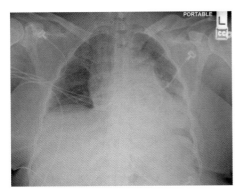

Figure 79.1

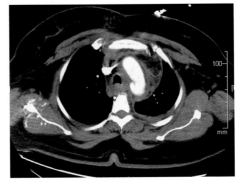

Figure 79.2

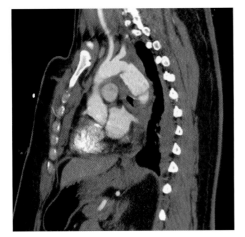

Figure 79.3

Case 79   Acute Traumatic Aortic Injury

Figure 79.4

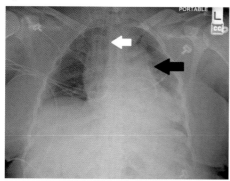

Figure 79.5

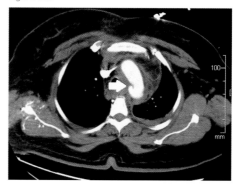

Figure 79.6

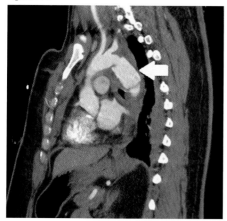

Figure 79.7

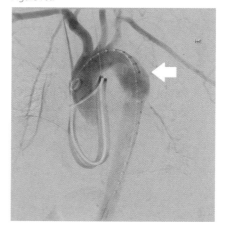

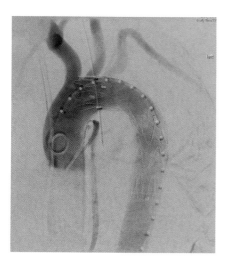

Figure 79.8

Findings

▶ Chest radiograph (Fig. 79.4) demonstrates a widened mediastinum (black arrow) and shift of the trachea to the right (white arrow). Depression of the left main bronchus may also be seen in the setting of traumatic aortic injury (not well depicted here).

▶ Axial and sagittal postcontrast images (Figs. 79.5 and 79.6) demonstrate disruption of the descending thoracic aorta just distal to the origin of the subclavian artery with associated contained pseudoaneurysm (white arrow).

▶ Figure 79.7 demonstrates the aortic injury on left anterior oblique aortic angiogram (white arrow) prior to successful endovascular repair (Fig. 79.8).

Teaching Points

▶ Most (75%–80%) aortic injuries are associated with high-speed motor vehicle collisions.

▶ Immediate mortality is 80%–90%, with 60%–80% of those who reach the hospital surviving a definitive repair.

▶ Traumatic aortic injury occurs following acute deceleration at locations where the aortic is relatively immobile. These include the aortic root, at the diaphragmatic hiatus, and most commonly at the aortic isthmus (as was seen in this case), where the aorta is tethered by the ligamentum arteriosum.

Management

▶ Acute traumatic aortic injury is a surgical emergency. Most patients undergo open surgical repair with aortic cross-clamping and cardiopulmonary bypass.

▶ Select cases, such as the one shown, can be treated with endovascular techniques depending on the degree and location of the injury as delineated on a contrast-enhanced computed tomography (CT) and immediate availability of appropriate size stent grafts.

Further Reading

Steenburg SD, Ravenel JG, Ikonomidis JS, et al. Acute traumatic aortic injury: imaging evaluation and management. *Radiology.* 2008; 248:748–762.

History

▶ A 50-Year-Old Male with Persistent Hypertension Despite Being Treated with Three Antihypertensive Medications

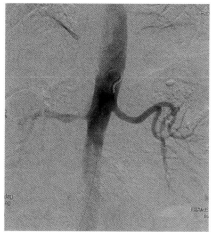

Figure 80.1

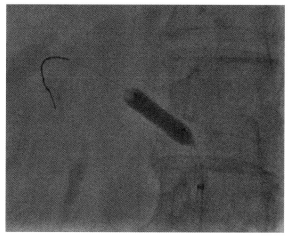

Figure 80.2

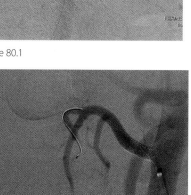

Figure 80.3

Case 80 Renal Artery Stenosis

Figure 80.4

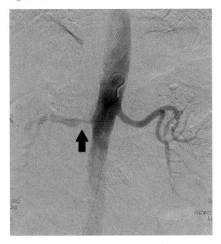

Figure 80.5

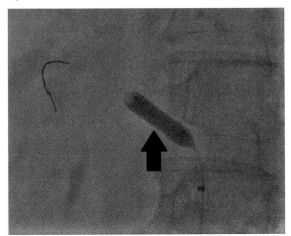

Figure 80.6

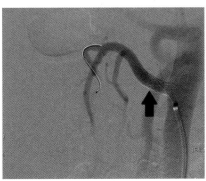

Findings

▶ Nonselective aortogram demonstrates a high-grade stenosis involving the right renal ostium (Fig. 80.4, arrow).

▶ Figure 80.5 shows deployment of a balloon expandable stent (arrow) across the ostial stenosis. Use of balloon expandable stents offers more precise deployment.

▶ Figure 80.6 shows a technically successful deployment of the stent (arrow). Blood pressure normalization occurred later that evening.

Teaching Points

▶ Renal artery stenosis (RAS) is a relatively common disease with a mortality rate of approximately 16%.

▶ While many patients are asymptomatic, this diagnosis should be considered in patients presenting with uncontrollable or abrupt onset of hypertension, hypertension with asymmetric renal length, and less commonly, flash pulmonary edema. If onset of hypertension occurs in a young person (<30 years of age), fibromuscular dysplasia should be considered.

▶ RAS results in activation with release of renin from renal juxtaglomerular cells. Renin catalyzes the breakdown of angiotensinogen to angiotensin I. Angiotensin I is transformed by angiotensin-converting enzyme into angiotensin II; and angiotensin II, a potent vasoconstrictor, promotes the release of aldosterone from the adrenal cortex.

- RAS is suggested to cause two types of hypertension:
  - Unilateral RAS with a normally perfused and normally functioning contralateral kidney; hypertension is referred to as "renin dependent" and is characterized by increased peripheral resistance. Renin and angiotensin levels are elevated, but volume expansion is limited by natriuresis of the contralateral normally functioning kidney.
  - Bilateral RAS or unilateral RAS with absent or dysfunctional contralateral kidney; intravascular volume increases and renin secretion decreases. Without the natriuretic effect of a normally perfused contralateral kidney, hypertension is maintained by volume expansion.
- Primary stenting is generally reserved for ostial lesions.

Management

- Use of renal artery angioplasty/stenting for treatment of hypertension is highly controversial, secondary to reports of no clinical benefit despite technical success. This may be secondary to poor patient selection and overtreatment. Thus, strict adherence to guidelines is suggested. Guidelines for renal artery revascularization suggest that a hemodynamically significant RAS is defined as the presence of $\geq$50% to 70% diameter stenosis by visual estimation on angiography, a systolic pressure gradient $\geq$20 mmHg, or a mean gradient $\geq$ 10 mmHg measured with a $\leq$ 5 French catheter or a pressure guidewire.
- Blood pressure normalization can be quick and profound occurring within hours to days after the procedure. Close monitoring and titration of blood pressure medications is important.

Further Reading

Hirsch AT, Haskal ZJ, Hertzer NR, et al. Practice guidelines for the management of patients with peripheral arterial disease (lower extremity, renal, mesenteric and abdominal aortic). *Circulation.* 2006; 113:e463–e654.

Case 81

History

▸ Right Groin Swelling and Pain 2 Weeks after Cardiac Catheterization

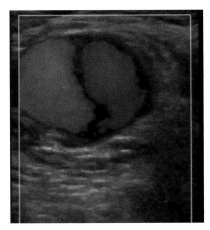

Figure 81.1

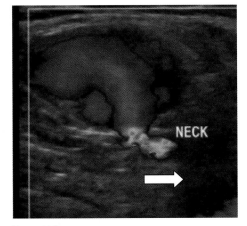

Figure 81.2

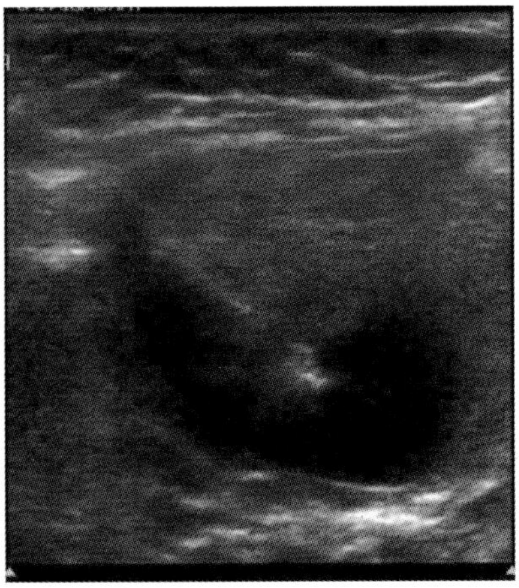

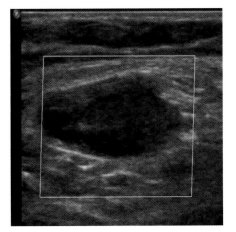

Figure 81.3

Figure 81.4

Case 81 Femoral Artery Pseudoaneurysm

Figure 81.5

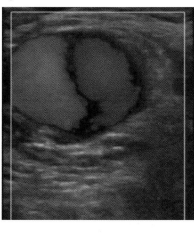

Figure 81.6

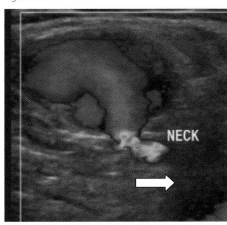

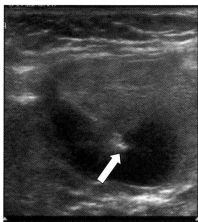

Figure 81.7

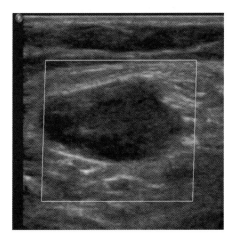

Figure 81.8

Findings

▶ Ultrasound of the groin demonstrates a right femoral artery pseudoaneurysm with a class "yin-yang" appearance of to-fro flow within (Fig. 81.5) and a narrow neck (Fig. 81.6) between the pseudoaneurysm and common femoral artery (arrow).

▶ A 22-gauge needle was advanced into the pseudoaneurysm (Fig. 81.7, arrow) under ultrasound guidance away from the neck.

▶ After injection of 1000 units of thrombin injection (Fig. 81.8) the pseudoaneurysm has completely thrombosed with no residual flow seen in the pseudoaneurysm sac.

Teaching Points

▶ After catheterization of the common femoral artery, the risk of pseudoaneurysm is approximately 2%.

▶ Risk factors include arterial puncture above the inguinal ligament or below the femoral head, use of anticoagulation, large sheaths, and female sex. Femoral access should be performed at the level of the femoral head because the hard bone acts as a back stop for manual compression of the artery.

▶ Swelling, pain, or a bruit at the site of an arterial puncture should raise the possibility of pseudoaneurysm. The diagnosis is made by ultrasound, which can demonstrate both anatomy and flow characteristics.

Management

▶ Small, asymotomatic pseudoaneurysms (<2 cm) may be managed conservatively with follow-up ultrasound in 2–4 weeks to confirm resolution.

▶ Treatment options include percutaneous thrombin injection, ultrasound-guided compression, and surgical repair.

▶ Ultrasound-guided compression involves compression with the ultrasound probe using enough pressure to collapse the pseudoaneurysm but to allow flow in the parent femoral artery. After 20 minutes, the pressure is released and flow within the lesion is reassessed. This may be repeated several times, but it is difficult for both the operator and patient to tolerate.

▶ Thrombin injection, when technically feasible, is performed by injection of small volumes (usually <1 cc) of 1,000 IU/mL topical thrombin as far from the neck as possible under constant ultrasound guidance. Care should be taken to avoid overinjection, which can result in thrombosis of the parent vessel.

Further Reading

Tisi PV, Callam MJ. Treatment for femoral pseudoaneurysms. *Cochrane Database Syst Rev.* 2013; 11:CD004981.

History

▶ A 78-Year-Old Female with History of Atrial Fibrillation and Acute Abdominal Pain

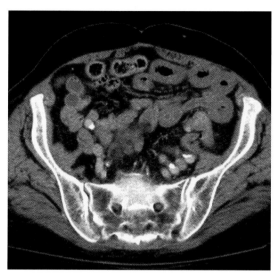

Figure 82.1

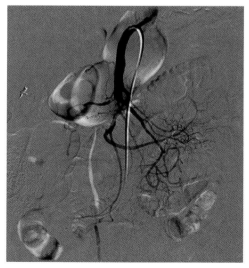

Figure 82.2

Case 82 Acute Superior Mesenteric Artery Embolism

Figure 82.3

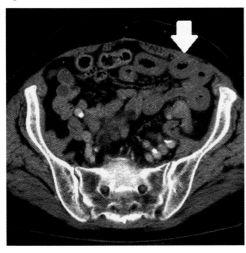

Figure 82.4

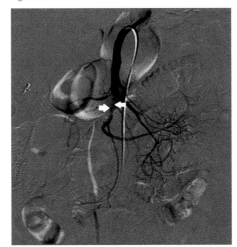

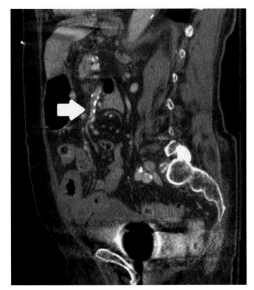

Figure 82.5

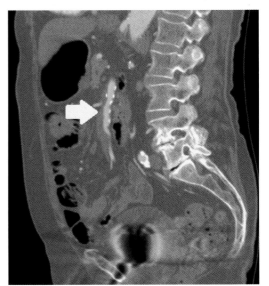

Figure 82.6

Findings

▶ Figure 82.3 demonstrates thickening of small-bowel loops in the mid-abdomen (white arrow). This finding is nonspecific but suggestive of an inflammatory or ischemic process.

▶ Figure 82.4 depicts a superior mesenteric angiogram with a filling defect (white arrows) in an intestinal branch of the superior mesenteric artery (SMA) supplying distal jejunal branches.

▶ Figure 82.5 is a sagittal computed tomography (CT) scan reconstructed from the scan from Figure 82.3. In retrospect, this filling defect may have been identified (white arrow); however, the phase of contrast injection and calcium makes the diagnosis difficult.

▶ Follow-up CT angiogram 6 months after emergent open thrombectomy and vein patch demonstrating a patent jejunal branch (Fig. 82.6, white arrow).

Teaching Points

► SMA embolism is the most common cause of acute mesenteric ischemia. Sudden obstruction of the celiac or inferior mesenteric artery is a rare cause of acute symptoms.

► Arteriography can be performed if findings on noninvasive imaging are equivocal, if nonocclusive ischemia is suspected, or if endovascular therapy is planned.

► Acute SMA embolism is best treated with surgical embolectomy with or without patch angioplasty or bypass grafting. This allows for evaluation of bowel viability and resection of infarcted bowel, if needed. In select cases without evidence of threatened bowel, thrombolysis may be considered.

► Vasodilator infusion (Papaverine) may be considered as a preoperative therapy in cases of nonocclusive embolism.

► Emboli typically lodge at branch points within the vessel and cause abrupt cutoff with a meniscus or tram-track appearance of contrast around the clot.

Management

► The most common source of acute mesenteric embolism is cardiac. In this case, left atrial thrombus due to atrial fibrillation was the culprit.

► Workup for cause of any embolic disease requires an evaluation for the source. In the case of visceral emboli, the workup should include an echocardiogram and possibly a CT angiogram of the aorta to exclude aneurysm as a source.

Further Reading

Ryer EJ, Kalra M, Oderich GS, et al. Revascularization for acute mesenteric ischemia. *Jour Vas Surg.* 2012; 55:1682–1689.

History

▶ A 35-Year-Old Female Presenting with Menorrhagia

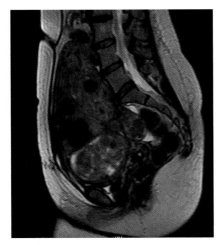

Figure 83.1

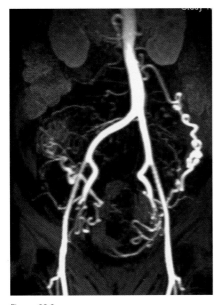

Figure 83.2

Case 83 Uterine Fibroid Embolization

Figure 83.3

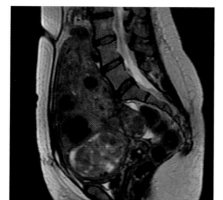

Figure 83.4

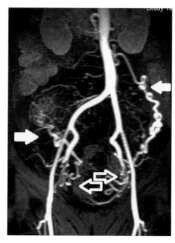

Figure 83.5

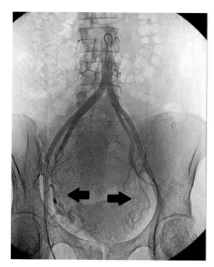

Figure 83.6

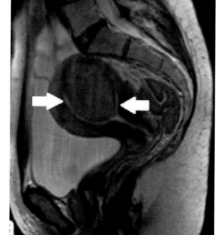

Findings

▶ Figure 83.3 demonstrates an enlarged uterus with multiple fibroids, some of which demonstrate internal cystic changes.

▶ Magnetic resonance angiogram (MRA) demonstrating enlarged uterine arteries (Fig. 83.4, open white arrows) and enlarged ovarian arteries (solid white arrows) supplying the hypervascular fibroids. Because of this finding, the patient was counseled that initial embolization may be suboptimal secondary to collateral supply from the ovarian vessels.

▶ Intraprocedural angiogram (Fig. 83.5) demonstrates enlarged uterine arteries (black arrows). Both right and left uterine arteries were selectively catheterized and embolized with spherical particles.

▶ Figure 83.6 is a companion image from a different patient demonstrating a submucosal fibroid with large intracavitary component (white arrows). Findings like this on a preprocedural magnetic resonance image (MRI) should prompt discussion of risk of postembolization infection and passage of necrotic tissue.

Teaching Points

▶ MR evaluation should be used to evaluate patients for candidacy and for follow-up after uterine fibroid embolization (UFE). Attention should be paid to the following:

  ▪ Intracavitary fibroids are likely to be expelled in weeks to months after a UFE, which may require antibiotics, analgesia, or assisted expulsion by a gynecologist.

  ▪ Pedunculated subserosal fibroids are considered a relative contraindication for embolization secondary to risk of detachment. Recent literature seems to suggest its safety; however, most practitioners are still cautious.

  ▪ Cervical fibroids may be resistant to UFE secondary to rich collateral blood supply.

▶ Contraindications to UFE include current uterine or adnexal infection, pregnancy, and suspected gynecologic malignancy.

▶ While controversial, UFE should not be considered first-line treatment for women with infertility secondary to fibroids or who desire to become pregnant, with studies suggesting myomectomy offering better outcomes.

Management

▶ Pain management plays an important role in the postprocedure setting with most patients receiving intravenous narcotics via a patient-controlled analgesia pump overnight.

▶ Most patients are discharged home the following day with oral analgesics, with pain expected to continue for about 1 week.

▶ Postembolization syndrome is expected 3–5 days after the procedure, comprised of low-grade fevers, generalized fatigue, and loss of appetite.

Further Reading

Bulman JC, Ascher SM, Spies JB. Current concepts in uterine fibroid embolization. *Radiographics* 2012; 32:1735–1750.

History

▶ A 30-Year-Old Male Runner with New-Onset Bilateral Calf Claudication

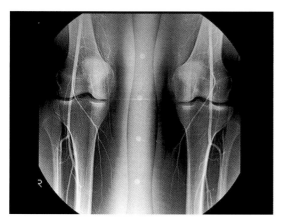

Figure 84.1

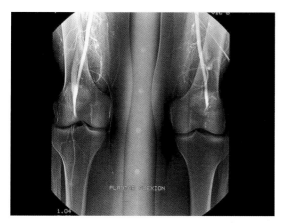

Figure 84.2

Case 84 Popliteal Entrapment

Figure 84.3

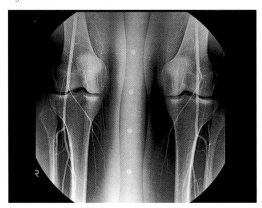

Figure 84.4

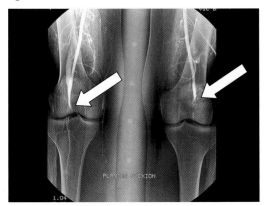

Findings

► Lower extremity arteriogram (Fig. 84.3) in neutral position of the ankle demonstrates normal flow and runoff of the bilateral popliteal arteries to the anterior tibial artery and tibioperoneal trunk.

► In plantar flexion (arrows, Fig. 84.4) there is abrupt occlusion of the left popliteal artery and significantly decreased runoff to the right calf.

Teaching Points

► Popliteal artery entrapment syndrome presents with calf claudication exacerbated with exercise. On physical examination distal pulses that decrease with plantar flexion should raise the possibility of entrapment.

► Anatomic popliteal entrapment is characterized by deviation and compression of the artery by the medial head of the gastrocnemius that can result in adventitial thickening, fibrosis, aneurysm formation, thrombosis, and distal embolization ("blue toe syndrome").

► Popliteal entrapment is bilateral in 20%–60% of cases and is most common in young and middle-aged patients.

► In functional popliteal entrapment, there is a normal anatomic relationship of the popliteal artery as it exits the popliteal fossa and passes between the medial and lateral heads of the gastrocnemius muscle and posterior to the popliteus muscle. In this situation, it is hypertrophy of the normally positioned calf muscles that results in compression of the artery during exercise.

Treatment

► With entrapment, the popliteal artery may appear normal in neutral position. Compression with plantar flexion clinches the diagnosis.

► Surgical release of the muscle or tendon is necessary for anatomic entrapment. There is no role for angioplasty or stent.

► Thrombolysis can be performed prior to surgery in patients who present with occlusion or emboli.

Further Reading

Wright LB, Matchett WJ, Cruz CP, et al. Popliteal artery disease: diagnosis and treatment. *Radiographics* 2004; 24(2):467–479.
    Acknowledgments
Images courtesy of Jim Caridi, MD, University of Florida, Gainesville, FL.

History

▶ Colon Cancer with Limited Liver Metastases Preoperative Right Trisegmentectomy

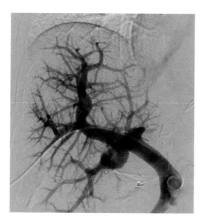

Figure 85.1

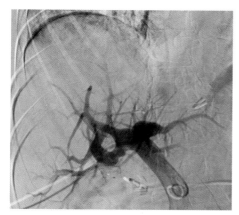

Figure 85.2

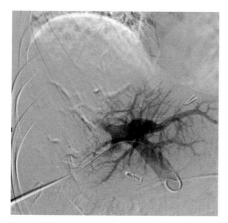

Figure 85.3

Case 85 Portal Vein Embolization

Figure 85.4

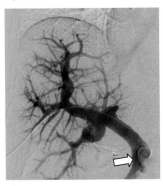

Figure 85.5

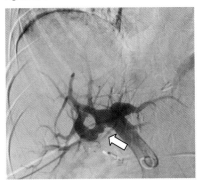

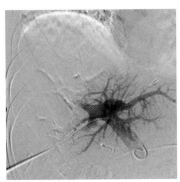

Figure 85.6

Findings

▶ Transhepatic access to the right posterior portal vein has been achieved, and a pigtail catheter is positioned in the main portal vein (Fig. 85.4, arrow).

▶ Portal venogram in the AP (Fig. 85.4) and RAO (Fig. 85.5) projections demonstrates aberrant portal vein branching pattern. The right posterior portal vein (arrow) is the first branch of the main portal vein in this so-called "Z-type" anatomy.

▶ Following embolization of the right portal vein (Fig. 85.6), there is redirection of flow to the future liver remanant (FLR), in this case the left hemiliver.

Teaching Points

▶ The indication for portal vein embolization is to induce contralateral hepatic hypertrophy to facilitate extended hepatic resection.

▶ Assessment of liver function may be functional or anatomic. Clearance of indocyanine green is an example of functional assessment and is commonly used preoperatively in Asia. Liver volumetric analysis, an anatomic measure, is more commonly used in the United States to assess resectability.

▶ Approximately 40% of patients have variant portal vein anatomy. This is important to recognize to prevent embolization of nontarget vessels and ensure embolization of all target branches.

Management

▶ In this case, embolization was performed with Embospheres©, although many agents can be used, including particles, glue, and thrombin. Coils are generally not used as a single agent because of the rich intrahepatic collaterals that reconstitued distal portal vein branches, but they may be used in combination with another agent.

▶ In patients with compensated cirrhosis, an FLR of 40% is considered adequate, whereas in patients with normal liver parenchyma an FLR of 20%–25% may be acceptable.

▶ Hypertrophy is commonly assessed by computed tomography or magnetic resonance volumetry 4 weeks after embolization. Typical increase in the ratio of future liver remnent/total liver volume is 8%–10% and the mean hypertrophy of the FLR is 25%–30%. In patients with cirrhosis the hypertrophy is less pronounced.

▶ Ipsilateral portal vein access is preferred to minimize the risk of damage to the FLR.

Further Reading

Avritscher R, de Baere T, Murthy R, et al. Percutaneous transhepatic portal vein embolization: rationale, technique, and outcomes. *Semin Intervent Radiol.* 2008; 25(2):132–145.

Covey AM, Brody LA, Getrajdman GI, et al. The incidence, patterns and clinical relevance of variant portal vein anatomy. *Am J Roentgenol.* 2004; 183(4):1055–1064.

History

▶ A 31-Year-Old Asian Female with History of Crohn's Disease and Sickle Cell Trait with Multiple Past Hospitalizations for Chest Pain and Myalgia

Multiple prior chest computed tomographs (CTs) performed were all negative. Recently, the patient was admitted with acute chest pain with the following imaging; findings are new since 6 months prior. Of note, the patient had previously been on chronic steroid therapy.

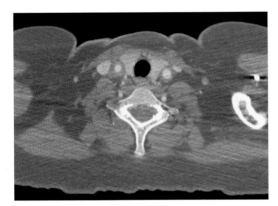

Figure 86.1

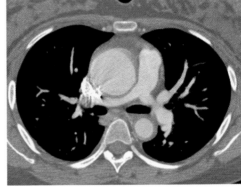

Figure 86.2

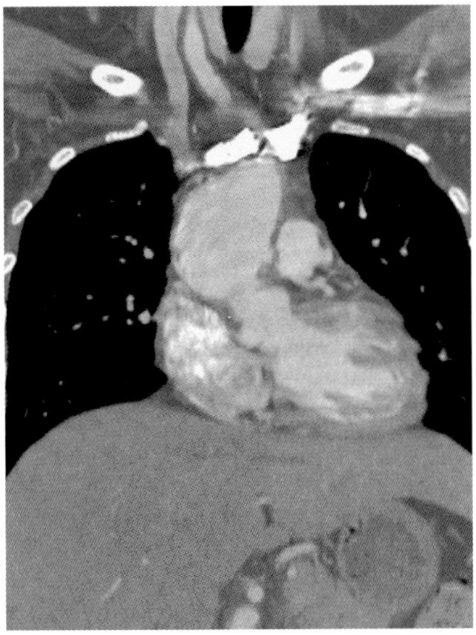

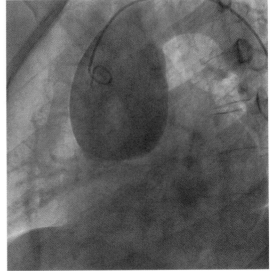

Figure 86.3

Figure 86.4

Case 86   Takayasu's Arteritis with Ascending Aortic Aneurysm

Figure 86.5

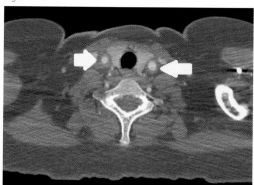

Figure 86.6

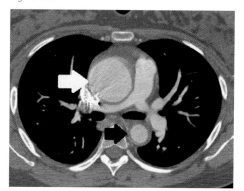

Figure 86.7

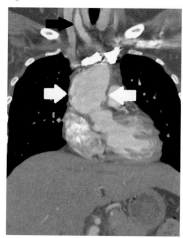

Figure 86.8

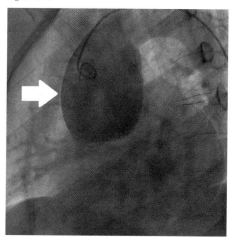

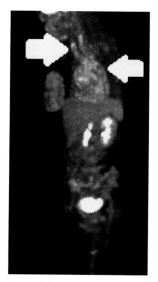

Figure 86.9

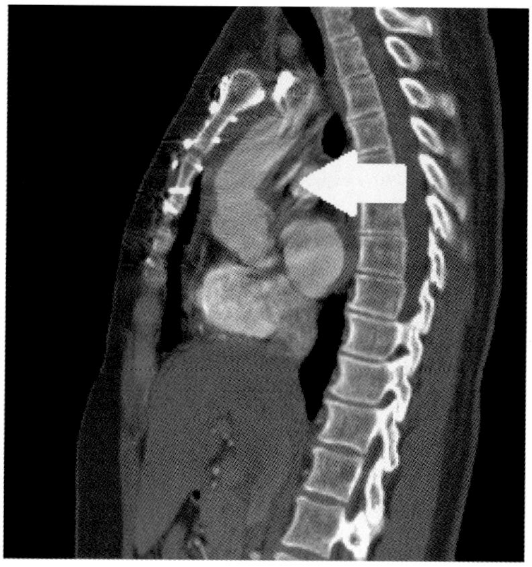

Figure 86.10

Findings

▸ CT scan on admission shows asymmetric stenosis of the right carotid artery with thickening of the arterial wall (white arrows, Fig. 86.4). Additionally, an ascending aortic aneurysm is identified (white arrows, Figs. 86.6 and 86.7), which was not seen on prior CT scans from 6 months prior (not shown). Thickening of the walls of the descending aorta (black arrow, Fig. 86.6) and carotid artery (black arrow, Fig. 86.5) are also identified.

▸ Figure 86.8 represents an ascending aortic angiogram showing a tulip bulb appearance of the ascending aorta (white arrow). Taken alone, this could also reflect aortic dilation from Marfan's syndrome; however, it is compatible with sequela of large-vessel vasculitis, given the remainder of findings on the corresponding CT.

▸ Active vasculitis is demonstrated as fluorodeoxyglucose (FDG) avidity on positron emission tomography (PET) imaging (white arrows, Fig. 86.9).

▸ Figure 86.10 shows 1-year follow-up after ascending aortic aneurysm repair (white arrow).

Teaching Points

▸ Takayasu's arteritis is an uncommon large-vessel vasculitis that can produce both stenosis and aneuryms. It is more common in females.

▸ It is considered an autoimmune disease, but it is thought to have a multifactorial etiology.

▸ Classical presentation includes two phases: an acute (prepulseless) phase and a late (pulseless) phase.
  ▪ Acute symptoms: often constitutional—weight loss, fatigue, night sweats, and fevers. May also include joint pain and arthritis.
  ▪ Late symptoms: usually secondary to organ involvement such as upper-extremity claudication, cerebrovascular insufficiency, or carotid artery pain.

▸ While nonspecific, inflammatory markers such as ESR and C-reactive protein may be elevated.

▸ Magnetic resonance imaging (MRI) or CT will show vessel wall thickening, stenosis, and/or aneurysm formation.

▸ PET/CT has been suggested to monitor signs of inflammation within the vessel wall.

▸ Current classification of Takayasu's arteritis is as follows, based on artery involvement:
  ▪ Type I—Arch vessels
  ▪ Type IIA—Ascending aorta, arch, and branches
  ▪ Type IIB—Type IIA + descending aorta
  ▪ Type III—Descending and abdominal aorta and/or renal artery
  ▪ Type IV—Abdominal aorta and renal artery
  ▪ Type V—Combination of types IIB and IV

Management

▸ Main therapy is medical with a combination of steroids and/or immunosuppressive drugs. Long-term prednisolone therapy can result in imaging improvement. Patients in the active phase are treated with a steroid taper.

▸ Surgery for symptomatic stenosis or enlarging aneurysms should only be performed after multidisciplinary discussion and avoided during the active phase.

▸ Intervention during the active phase is associated with poor outcome. In the latent phase, angioplasty to treat chronic stenosis can be considered. There are scattered reports of endograft placement to treat aneurysmal components.

Further Reading

Gotway MB, Araz PA, Macedo TA, et al. Imaging findings in Takayasu's arteritis. *Am J Roentgenol*. 2005; 184:1945–1950.

Tombetti E, Manfredi A, Sabbadini MG, et al. Management options for Takayasu arteritis. *Expert Opin on Orphan Drug*. 2013; 1:685–693.

History

▶ A 69-Year-Old Diabetic Male with Atherosclerosis and Upper Thigh/Buttock Claudication

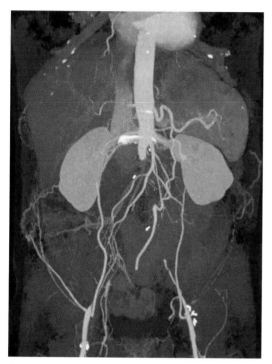

Figure 87.1

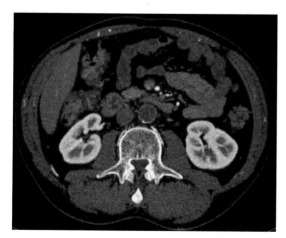

Figure 87.2

Case 87 Leriche Syndrome

Figure 87.3

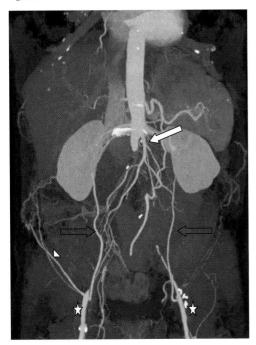

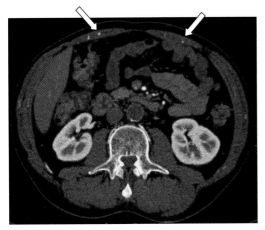

Figure 87.4

Findings

▶ MIP from a contrast-enhanced magnetic resonance image (MRI) (Fig. 87.3) demonstrates abrupt cutoff of the abdominal aorta just below the origin of the superior mesenteric artery (arrow). The external iliac arteries (stars) are reconstituted by collaterals, including prominent inferior epigastric arteries (hollow arrows) and iliolumbar arteries (arrowhead).

▶ Arterial-phase axial contrast-enhanced computed tomography (CT) (Fig. 87.4) confirms complete occlusion of the distal aorta and shows large inferior epigastric arteries (arrows) that serve as a collateral pathway to reconstitute the external iliac arteries.

Teaching Points

▶ The constellation of bilateral buttock claudication, impotence (in men), and diminished femoral pulses is termed "Leriche syndrome." Symptoms may be unilateral or bilateral, depending on the level of obstruction and efficacy of collateral pathways.

▶ Leriche syndrome occurs in the setting of atherosclerotic aortoiliac occlusive disease usually distal to origin of the renal arteries. This is a differentiating factor from mid-aortic syndrome, which is seen in children and young adults and involves the origins of the renal arteries.

▶ Collateral pathways that provide lower-extremity runoff in the setting of aortoiliac occlusive disease include (1) the "Winslow pathway" from the internal mammary or intercostal arteries to the external iliac arteries via the inferior epigastric arteries (as in this case); (2) lumbar to iliolumbar arteries; (3) superior hemorrhoidal (a branch of the inferior mesenteric artery) to inferior hemorrhoidal arteries; and (4) various additional communications between branches of the internal iliac artery and femoral arteries (e.g., superior gluteal to femoral circumflex).

Management

▶ Diagnostic catheter angiography is rarely indicated because CT angiogram and magnetic resonance angiogram can provide the morphologic and physiologic information required to plan intervention.

▶ Indications for intervention include disabling claudication and threatened limb.

▶ Surgical options include aortofemoral bypass, axillofemoral bypass, femoral-femoral bypass, and aortic endarterectomy.

▶ In some cases, stent placement can be performed, with the best results in single lesions <3 cm; however, this is an uncommon cause of Leriche syndrome.

Further Reading

Hardman RL, Lopera JE, Cardan RA, et al. Common and rare collateral pathways in aortoiliac occlusive disease: a pictorial essay. *Am J Roentgenol.* 2011; 197(3):W519–W524.

Kaufman J, Lee MJ. Abdominal aorta and iliac arteries. In: *Vascular and Interventional Radiology: The Requisites.* Elsevier-Mosby; 2004:261–270.

History

▶ A 40-Year-Old Female Who Presents with Sudden Onset of Blue Fingers

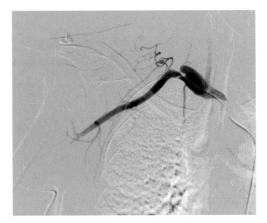

Figure 88.1

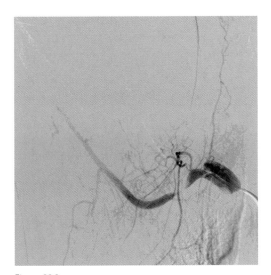

Figure 88.2

Case 88 Thoracic Outlet Syndrome and Subclavian Artery Aneurysm

Figure 88.3

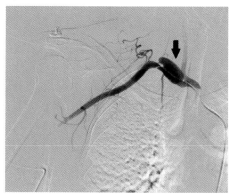

Figure 88.4

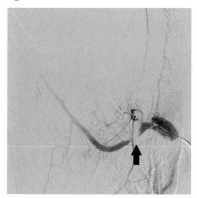

Findings

▶ A selective arteriogram of the right subclavian artery in neutral position (Fig. 88.3) shows a large aneurysm (black arrow) involving the proximal right subclavian artery. This aneurysm is the source of emboli causing blue fingers.

▶ Repeated arteriogram of the right subclavian artery with the arm abducted (Fig. 88.4) shows compression of the subclavian artery (black arrow) at the thoracic outlet. Aneurysms secondary to thoracic outlet compression usually occur just proximal to the area of compression, making this case atypical.

Teaching Points

▶ Thoracic outlet syndrome refers to compression of the neurovascular bundle by either normal or variant anatomical structures. Commonly, these include the first rib, the anterior scalene muscle, an anomalous cervical rib, or the tendon of the subclavius muscle.

▶ Physical exam may reveal arm pain, skin color changes, or muscle cramping during abduction of the affected limb.

▶ Sonography may reveal increased peak systolic velocities or cessation of flow when the arm is placed in the hyperabducted position.

▶ To clinch the diagnosis of thoracic outlet syndrome at angiography, injections should be performed in both a neutral and abducted position to assess anatomy, severity of compression, and associated findings such as aneurysm formation or distal emboli.

Management

▶ Surgical release of the thoracic outlet should be performed prior to any endovascular therapy, except in the setting of limb ischemia or thrombus/emboli, where catheter-directed thrombolysis may be performed prior to surgical resection.

▶ Endovascular stent graft placement has been used to exclude aneurysms following surgical release; however, vascular bypass with aneurysm exclusion and resection may be required.

▶ Postsurgical angiography is performed to assess for residual stenosis, which may require further therapy.

▶ The patient in this case underwent first-rib resection with excision of the aneurysm with interposition graft.

Further Reading

Criado E, Berguer R, Greenfield L. The spectrum of arterial compression at the thoracic outlet. *J Vasc Surg*. 2010; 52:406–411.
Demondion X, Herbinet P, Van Sint Jan S, et al. Imaging assessment of thoracic outlet syndrome. *Radiographics*. 2006; 26:1735–1750.

History

▶ Neuroendocrine Liver Metastases. What is the Finding on the CT confirmed on the Angiogram?

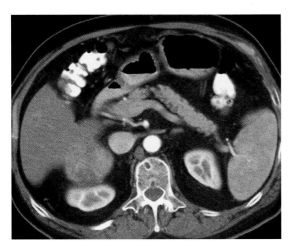

Figure 89.1

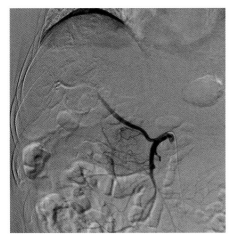

Figure 89.2

Case 89 Variant Hepatic Arterial

Figure 89.3

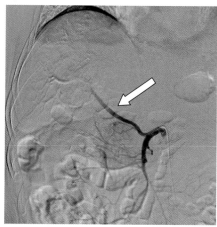

Figure 89.4

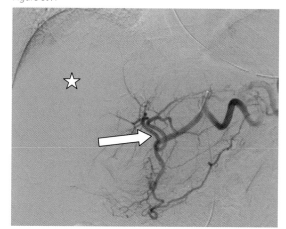

Figure 89.5

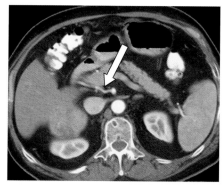

Figure 89.6

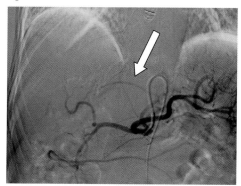

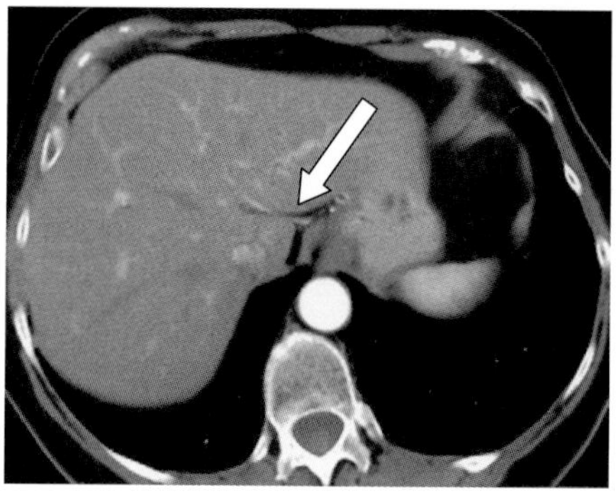

Figure 89.7

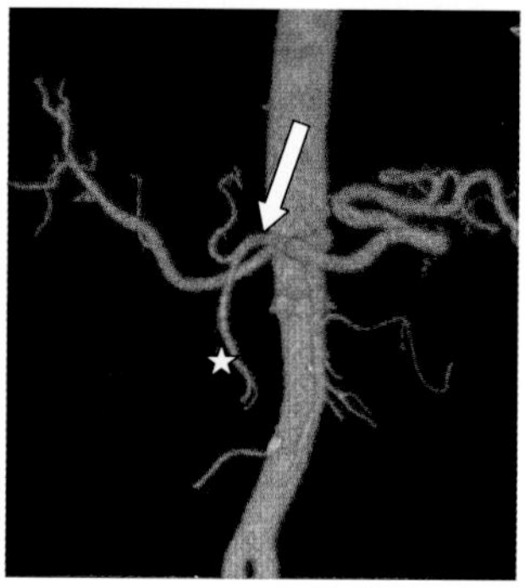

Figure 89.8

Findings

▶ Contrast enhanced axial CT image (Fig. 89.1) shows a vessel arising from a the superior mesenteric artery (SMA) and coursing between the portal vein and inferior vena cava. Catheter angiography confirms the first branch of SMA is a replaced right hepatic artery (Fig. 89.3).

▶ Celiac angiogram in a different patient (Fig. 89.4) with the same anatomy demonstrates the left hepatic artery (arrow) and no artery to the right hemiliver (star) arising from the common hepatic artery.

- In a different patient, celiac angiogram shows a vessel arising from the left gastric artery (Fig. 89.6, arrow) supplying the left hemiliver.
- The corresponding CT (Fig. 89.7) shows the replaced left hepatic artery arising from the left gastric artery (arrow).
- Figure 89.8 is a reconstruction from a CT angiogram demonstrating an uncommon variant, a double hepatic artery, in which the right and left hepatic arteries arise separately from the proximal celiac artery. In this case the gastroduodenal artery (star) is a branch of the left hepatic artery (arrow).

Teaching Points

- Replaced or accessory hepatic vessels are common, seen in approximately 40% of patients.
- The most common hepatic artery variant is an accessory left hepatic artery, followed by a replaced right hepatic artery (approximately 10% each). The term "accessory" refers to the situation in which only a part of the blood supply to a hemiliver is derived from the aberrant vessel.
- Recognition of variant anatomy is important for both surgeons contemplating liver and pancreatic surgery and interventional radiologists treating liver tumors or hemorrhage.
- On CT the differential diagnosis of soft tissue in the portocaval space includes a replaced right hepatic artery, papillary process of the caudate lobe, and enlarged lymph node(s).

Management

- Assessment of hepatic artery anatomy on preprocedure or preoperative imaging is an important part of the workup of patients undergoing hepatobiliary or pancreatic intervention in order to avoid either incomplete treatment when performing embolization or unanticipated intraoperative hemorrhage.

Further Reading

Covey Am, Brody LA, Maluccio MA, et al. Variant hepatic arterial anatomy revisited: digital subtraction angiography performed in 600 patients. *Radiology* 2002; 224:542–547.

History

▶ A 15-Year-Old Female with Progressive Right Lower-Extremity Pain

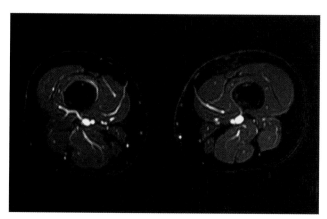

Figure 90.1

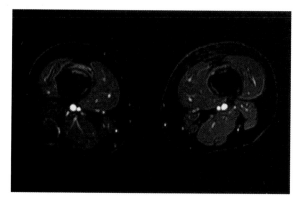

Figure 90.2

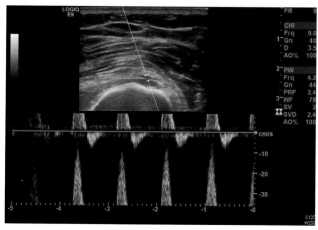

Figure 90.3

Case 90 Venous Malformation Sclerosis

Figure 90.4

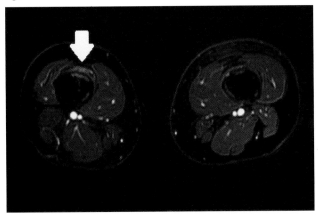

Figure 90.5

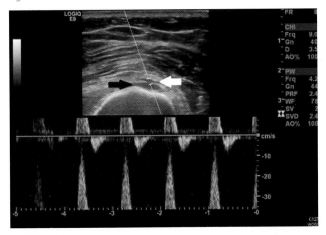

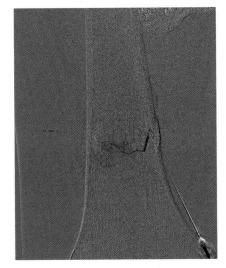

Figure 90.6

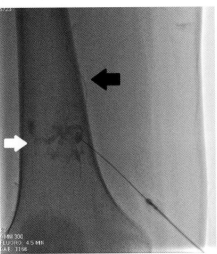

Figure 90.7

Findings

▶ Figure 90.4 demonstrates a T2 hyperintense venous malformation anterior to the right distal femur (white arrow) associated with a single feeding artery from the distal popliteal artery.

▶ Figures 90.5 shows the corresponding ultrasound demonstrating the feeding artery (white arrow) and associated malformation (black arrow).

▶ Figure 90.6 shows percutaneous access to the feeding artery.

▶ Figure 90.7 shows direct puncture of the nidus (white arrow) with associated draining vein (black arrow).

Teaching Points

▶ Vascular malformations are congenital lesions characterized by an inborn defect in various stages of embryogenesis involving one or a combination of arteries, veins, capillaries, or lymphatics.

▶ Vascular malformations are categorized into lymphatic malformations, low-flow venous malformations, or high-flow arteriovenous malformations (see Case 68).

Management

▶ Treatments are directed toward the malformation itself, not the arterial supply:
  ▪ First-line treatment of lymphatic or low-flow venous malformations includes direct puncture of the malformation and sclerosant injection.
  ▪ First-line treatment of a high-flow arteriovenous malformation involves percutaneous transarterial embolization.
  ▪ Sclerosants include ethanol, polidocanol, 3% sodium tetradecol sulfate (STS), and bleomycin, all with varying efficacy and complication profiles.

▶ Tourniquet use proximal to the treatment site should be considered to limit reflux on sclerosant into the normal venous system. A tourniquet was used during injection of the malformation shown in Figure 90.7 to increase dwell time of the sclerosant and to limit escape of sclerosant into the draining vein.

▶ Patients should be counseled on the likely need for multiple sessions of sclerosant injection spanned over weeks to months for complete treatment.

Further Reading

El-Merhi F, Garg D, Cura M, et al. Peripheral vascular tumors and vascular malformations: imaging (magnectic resonance imaging and conventional angiography), pathologic correlation and treatment options. *Int J Cardiovasc Imaging.* 2013; 29:379–393.

History

▶ A 70-Year-Old Male with "Drop Attacks"

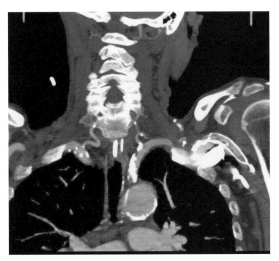

Figure 91.1

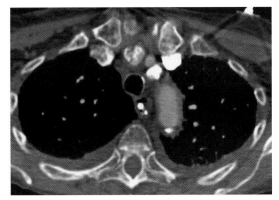

Figure 91.2

Case 91   Subclavian Steal

Figure 91.3

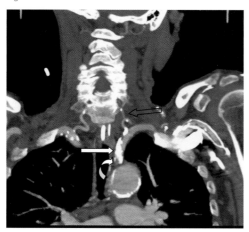

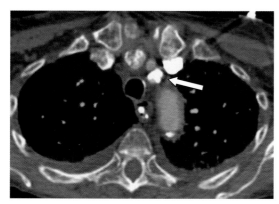

Figure 91.4

Findings

▶ Coronal (Fig. 91.3) and axial (Fig. 91.4) computed tomography (CT) following left upper-extremity contrast injection images show dense calcification of the origin of the left subclavian artery.

▶ No contrast is seen opacifying the origin of the subclavian artery; distal to the calcific occlusion there is reconstitution by retrograde flow in the left vertebral artery (hollow arrow).

Teaching Points

▶ "Subclavian steal" occurs when there is occlusion of a subclavian artery proximal to the origin of the vertebral artery. "Steal" results when retrograde flow in the ipsilateral vertebral artery provides the flow to the subclavian artery, resulting in decreased perfusion of the posterior cerebral circulation and syncope when the affected arm is exercised.

▶ Patients can also present with headaches, nausea, vertigo, ataxia, arm pain, paresthesias, and weakness. Vigorous exercise and a sudden sharp turning of the head in the direction of the affected side can also evoke symptoms.

▶ Contrast magnetic resonance (MR), computed tomography (CT), or Doppler ultrasound can be useful in making the diagnosis, but of the three, only Doppler ultrasound is truly dynamic and can measure differential flow during the cardiac cycle.

- Severity is classified by flow in the vertebral artery:
  - Grade 1 (presubclavian steal)—reduced antegrade vertebral flow
  - Grade 2 (intermittent/partial/latent)—retrograde flow in systole and antegrade flow in diastole
  - Grade 3 (permanent/advanced)—permanent retrograde vertebral flow
- Subclavian steal is most commonly due to atherosclerosis but can also be seen in patients with dissecting aneurysm, medium-vessel vasculitis (e.g., Takayasu arteritis), and radiation fibrosis.
- Signs on physical examination include weak or absent pulse or differential systolic pressure compared to the contralateral arm. In patients with left internal mammary coronary artery bypass grafts, symptoms can include cardiac ischemia.

Treatment

- Medical therapy is recommended for all patients with atherosclerotic disease, focusing on reducing the risk of atherosclerosis, including treating hypertension, hyperlipidemia, diabetes mellitus, and smoking cessation.
- Surgery and endovascular stent placement are indicated when symptoms of syncope, or coronary ischemia in the presence of a left internal mammary coronary artery bypass graft is present.

Further Reading

Burihan E, Soma F, Iared W. Angioplasty versus stenting for subclavian artery stenosis. *Cochrane Database Syst Rev.* 2011; (10):CD008461.

Ernemann U, Bender B, Melms A, et al. Current concepts of the interventional treatment of proximal supraaortic vessel stenosis. *Vasa.* 2012; 41(5):313–318.

History

▶ A 9-Year-Old Girl with Facial Swelling. What Are the Treatment Options?

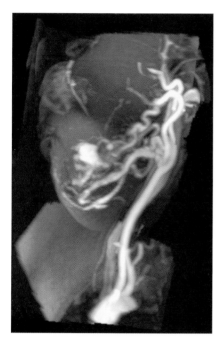

Figure 92.1

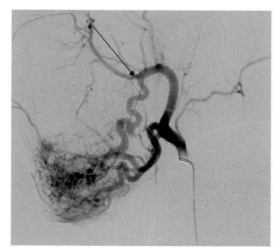

Figure 92.2

Case 92 Arteriovenous Malformation

Figure 92.3

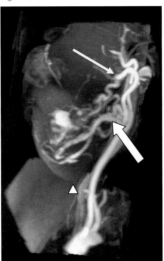

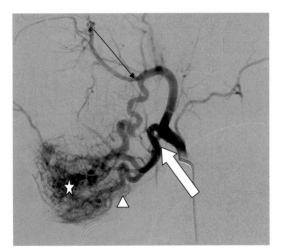

Figure 92.4

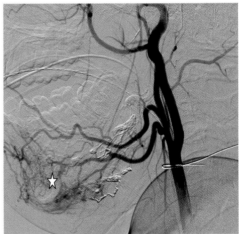

Figure 92.5

Findings

▶ MIP magnetic resonance image (MRI) (Fig. 92.3) shows an arteriovenous malformation (AVM) in the mandible with markedly enlarged branches of the internal maxillary artery (narrow arrow) and overlapped lingual and submental arteries (block arrow) with drainage into the jugular veins (arrowheads).

▶ Lateral view of a digital subtraction angiogram of the external carotid artery (Fig. 92.4) demonstrates the vascular nidus (star). Again noted are enlarged mandibular (small arrow), submental, and sublingual (arrow) feeding arteries.

▶ A combination of Onyx and coils was used to embolize the nidus and feeding vessels. Postembolization angiogram shows a decrease in the size of the nidus (star, Fig. 92.5).

Teaching Points

▶ AVMs consist of multiple dysplastic arteries that shunt directly into arterialized veins, creating a vascular nidus without a normal intervening capillary network.

▶ High-flow AVMs usually present in childhood. Periods of rapid growth are typically seen with growth spurts, puberty, and pregnancy.

▶ Syndromes associated with AVMs include hereditary hemorrhagic telengectasia and Parkes-Weber syndrome, which usually involves a lower extremity.

▶ The clinical staging system of AVMs based on the Schobinger Scale is as follows:

Stage I (Quiescence): cutaneous blush, skin warmth, arteriovenous shunt on Doppler ultrasound

Stage II (Expansion): darkening blush, lesion shows pulsation, thrill, and bruit

Stage III (Destruction): arterialsteal, distal ischemia, pain, dystrophic skin changes, ulceration, necrosis, soft tissue/bony changes

Stage IV (Decompensation): high-output cardiac failure

Treatment

▶ Most AVMs are inoperable or require extensive resection, which can be severely disfiguring.

▶ Destruction of the nidus is imperative to treating these difficult lesions. Simply embolizing the feeding arteries leads to recruitment of collateral vessels, which are typically a more circuitous route to accessing the nidus in the future.

▶ Percutaneous embolization can be used as primary treatment or as an adjunct to surgery. Complete eradication of the nidus can be extremely difficult, and repeat treatments are often necessary. Any one or a combination of ethanol, particles, tissue adhesives, nonadhesive liquid embolic agents (Onyx), and coils have been used.

▶ Particles should be avoided because they do not destroy the nidus and can pass into the venous outflow, resulting in paradoxical emboli.

▶ In this case, the patient underwent three embolizations of feeding vessels prior to surgery. The first two were with Onyx to decrease the size of the AVM. Final embolization was performed with coils to decrease intraoperative bleeding.

Acknowledgments

Images courtesy of Deborah Rabinowitz, MD, Alfred I. Dupont Children's Hospital, Wilmington, DE.

Further Reading

Cahill AM, Nijs EL. Pediatric vascular malformations: pathophysiology, diagnosis, and the role of interventional radiology. *Cardiovasc Intervent Radiol.* 2011; 34(4):691–704.

History

▶ Abdominal Pain and Fever

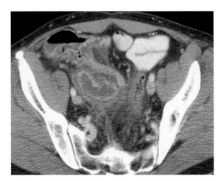

Figure 93.1

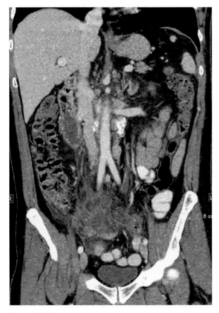

Figure 93.2

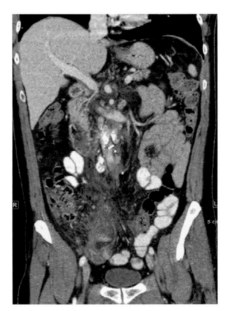

Figure 93.3

Case 93 Ruptured Appendix

Figure 93.4

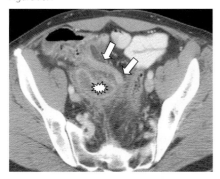

Figure 93.5

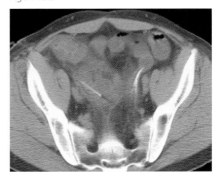

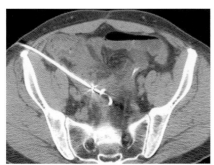

Figure 93.6

Findings

▶ Figure 93.4: There is a complex fluid collection in the right lower quadrant with an enhancing rim (star). A thickened appendix is identified immediately anterior to the collection (arrows).

▶ Anterior to the iliacus and posterior to the right colon, a 21-gauge needle has been advanced into the collection using computed tomography (CT) guidance (Fig. 93.5).

▶ A drainage catheter was placed into the collection (Fig. 93.6), and 25 cc of foul-smelling pus was aspirated. After placement of the catheter, there is minimal residual collection.

Teaching Points

▶ Perforated appendicitis may be drainage percutaneously prior to semielective appendectomy.

▶ Using CT guidance, drainage of the collection was performed even with a very narrow window of access. Other routes to collections deep in the pelvis include transgluteal, transpiriformis, transgluteal and approaches.

Management

▶ Antibiotics should be given within 1 hour of drainage of an abdominal abscess to minimize the risk of sepsis.

▶ Historically, drainage catheters were left in place until interval appendectomy was performed, but contemporary data suggest that in select cases conservative (nonoperative) management has fewer complications and similar reoperation rate to interval appendectomy.

Further Reading

Simillis C, Symeonides P, Shorthouse AJ, et al. A meta-analysis comparing conservative treatment versus acute appendectomy for complicated appendicitis (abscess or phlegmon). *Surgery* 2010; 147(6):818–829.

History

▶ A 50-Year-Old Female with Fevers and Leukocytosis 6 Days after Right Hemicolectomy

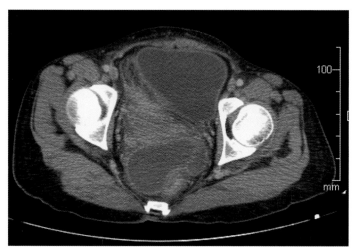

Figure 94.1

Case 94   Transgluteal Pelvic Abscess Drainage

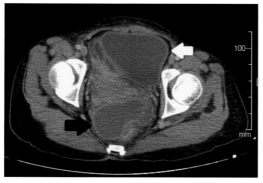

Figure 94.2

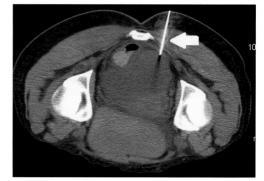

Figure 94.3

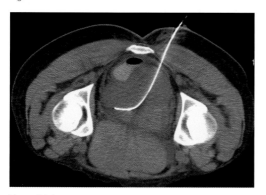

Figure 94.4

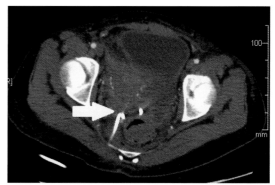

Figure 94.5

Findings

▶ An enhancing collection (black arrow) is seen the pelvis posterior to the urinary bladder (white arrow, Fig. 94.2) There is no safe route for transabdominal drainage, but the collection is amenable to transgluteal drainage.

▶ An access needle (Fig. 94.3, white arrow) is being advanced into the collection, taking care to be as close to the sacrum as possible. In this case, access below the piriformis and at the level of the sacrospinous ligament was used.

▶ Figure 94.4 shows the access wire within the collection prior to drain placement.

▶ Interval follow-up computed tomography (CT) (Fig. 94.5) shows near-complete resolution of the collection (white arrow).

Teaching Points

▶ Major neurovascular structures are located above the sacrospinous ligament, which marks the inferior border of the greater sciatic foramen.

▶ An approach inferior to the piriformis muscle is preferred to avoid risk of injury to the sacral plexus or gluteal vasculature.

▶ If entry to the collection is obscured by air in the distal sigmoid, consider placing a rectal tube to decompress.

▶ If an obvious route to the collection is not identified, consider techniques such as angling the CT gantry or hydrodissection.

▶ Pain radiating down the patient's leg during the procedure suggests that the needle is close to the sciatic nerve or a sacral nerve branch. The trajectory of the needle should be revised.

Management

▶ As with most abscess drains, catheter outputs are monitored daily and 10 cc forward flushes are performed 2–3 times daily, taking care to flush both the catheter entering the cavity and the tubing to the drainage bag.

▶ Removal of drain is considered once there is resolution of clinical and laboratory signs of infection.

▶ If there is persistent increased output in the drain, an enteric fistula should be suspected.

Further Reading

Harisinghani MG, Gervais DA, Hahn PF, et al. CT-guided transgluteal drainage of deep pelvic abscesses: indication, technique, procedure-related complications, and clinical outcome. *Radiographics*. 2002; 22:1353–1367.

History

▶ An 87-Year-Old Diabetic Male with Bladder Cancer, Fever, and Pelvic Pain. Where is the Abscess and What is the Most Appropriate Approach for Aspiration?

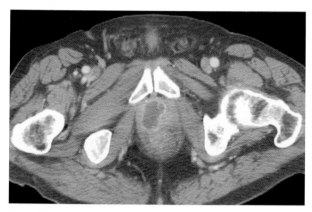

Figure 95.1

Case 95 Transrectal Aspiration of Prostatic Abscess

Figure 95.2

Figure 95.3

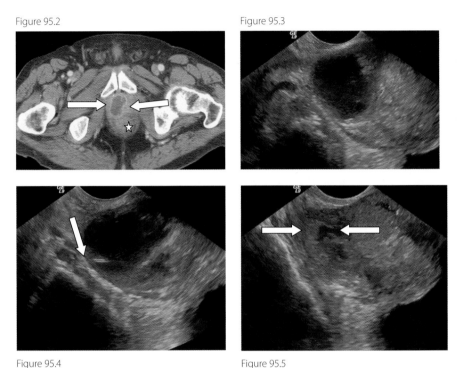

Figure 95.4

Figure 95.5

Findings

▶ Axial computed tomography (CT) (Fig. 95.2) shows a 3.2 cm rim enhancing collection within the inferior aspect of the prostate (arrows) gland just anterior to the rectum (star).

▶ Transrectal ultrasound (Fig. 95.3) demonstrates a nonloculated collection within the prostate corresponding to the finding on CT.

▶ Using transrectal ultrasound for guidance, a 20-gauge needle (Fig. 95.4, arrow) was advanced into the abscess under direct sonographic visualization.

▶ After 12 cc purulent fluid was aspirated, there is near complete resolution of the abscess cavity (Fig. 95.5, arrows).

Teaching Points

▶ Transrectal drainage is a reasonable treatment option in patients with deep pelvic or prostate abscesses not otherwise amenable to percutaneous (transgluteal/transperineal) drainage.

▶ Endocavitary drainage (transrectal, transvaginal) is surprisingly well tolerated by patients, and in some cases even for percutaneously accessible collections may be favorable to percutaneous drainage for this reason. This is especially the case in pediatric patients.

▶ Prostatic abscesses are usually seen in patients who have diabetes or other cause for immunosuppression who become inoculated from a urinary tract infection, indwelling urinary drainage catheter, or biopsy.

▶ Historically, prostatic abscesses were most commonly related to Neisseria gonorrhea. Current offending organisms are those related to urinary tract, including *Escherichia coli* and other gram-negative bacilli.

Management

▶ For periuretheral abscesses, transureteral prostate resection is an alternative treatment option.

▶ In some cases, a drain may be left in place for a short dwell time to maximize drainage.

Further Reading

Arrabal-Polo MA, Jimenez-Pacheco A, Arrabal-Martin M. Percutaneous drainage of prostatic abscess: case report and literature review. *Urol Int.* 2012; 88(1):118–120.

Sudakoff GS, Lundeen SJ, Otterson MF. Transrectal and transvaginal sonographic intervention of infected pelvic fluid collections: a complete approach. *Ultrasound Q.* 2005; 21(3):175–185.

History

▶ A 34-Year-Old Male Status Post Motor Vehicle Accident with Left Thigh Swelling

A drain was placed percutaneously in the collection noted in Figure 96.1. The drain remained for 2 weeks with persistent 30–40 cc daily serous-milky output. Figure 96.2 demonstrates a contrast study through the indwelling drain. What are the treatment options?

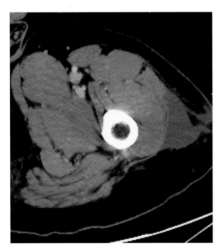

Figure 96.1

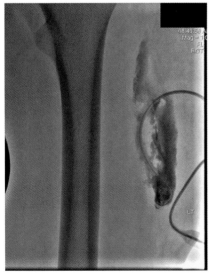

Figure 96.2

Case 96 Sclerosis of Traumatic Lymphocele

Figure 96.3

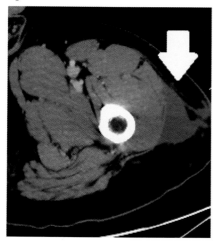

Figure 96.4

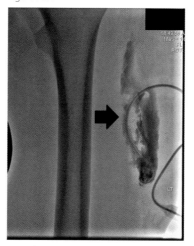

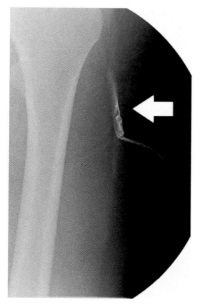

Figure 96.5

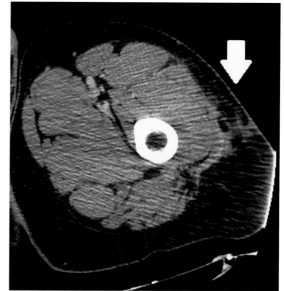

Figure 96.6

Findings

▶ A low-density fluid collection in the soft tissues of the lateral thigh (Fig. 96.3, white arrow).

▶ Contrast injection 2 weeks after initial drain placement (Fig. 96.4) was performed because of persistent outputs to determine cavity size (arrow). A total of 30 cc of contrast was required to completely opacify the cavity.

▶ After 2 weeks of daily povodine iodine sclerosis, there is near-complete resolution of the collection (Fig. 96.5, arrow). Only 2 cc of contrast could be injected prior to leakage out the drain tract. The drain was removed.

▶ CT was performed 1 week after drain removal, showing complete resolution of the collection (Fig. 96.6, white arrow).

Teaching Points

▶ Most lymphoceles are iatrogenic, related to pelvic or retroperitoneal surgery.
▶ There are various treatment options available to treat lymphoceles with persistent ranging from surgical marsupialization to catheter drainage to sclerotherapy.
▶ Many lymphoceles can be treated conservatively with spontaneous resolution.
▶ Lymphoceles can result in symptoms ranging from abdominal pain to urinary symptoms or constipation if they compresses on the urinary bladder or bowel, respectively. If compressing on venous structures, patients can also present with deep venous thrombosis.

Management

▶ Initial management may be aspiration or transcatheter drainage.
▶ Multiple sclerosants have been used for this purpose, the most common agents include ethanol, povidone iodine, doxycycline, and bleomycin with varying success. Local preferences apply. This author trials use of povidone iodine for 2–4 weeks, instructing the patient to inject the same volume as cavity size daily with a 1 hour dwell time for cavities up to 50 cc. Doxycycline, ethanol, or bleomycin may be useful for treating lymphoceles resistant to povidone iodine sclerosis.

Further Reading

Alago W, Deodhar A, Michell H, et al. Management of postoperative lymphoceles after lymphadenectomy: percutaneous catheter drainage with and without povidone-iodine sclerotherapy. *Cardiovasc Intervent Radiol.* 2013; 36:466–471.

Mahrer A, Ramchandani P, Trerotola SO, et al. Sclerotherapy in the management of postoperative lymphocele. *J Vasc Interv Radiol.* 2010; 21:1050–1053.

Case 97

History

- A 65-Year-Old Female with Gastric Cancer Who Developed an Anterior Abdominal Collection after Partial Gastrectomy Is Transferred to Your Care after Drainage with Persistent High Outputs

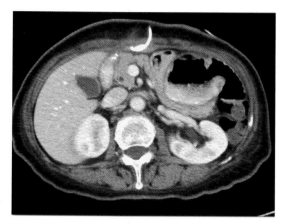

Figure 97.1

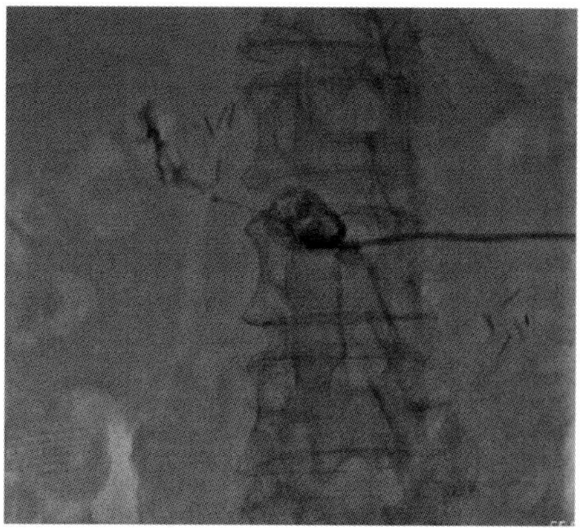

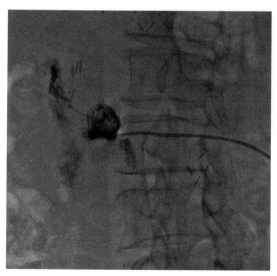

Figure 97.2

Figure 97.3

Case 97 Small-Bowel Fistula

Figure 97.4

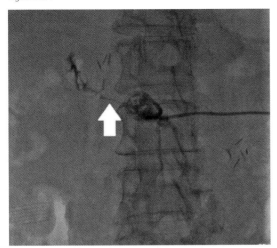

Figure 97.5

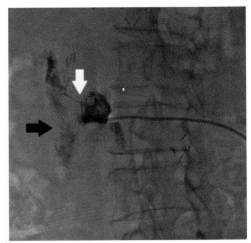

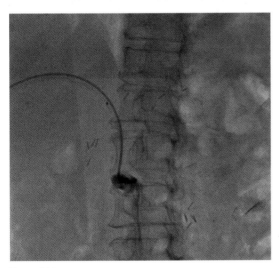

Figure 97.6

Findings

- A drainage catheter is seen in the anterior abdomen (Fig. 97.1). The collection that was drained (not shown) has near completely resolved.
- Contrast injection into the indwelling drainage catheter (Fig. 97.4) demonstrates a near completely resolved collection with a small sinus tract extending laterally (white arrow).
- A later image from the contrast injection (Fig. 97.5) shows increased filling of the structure now recognizable as duodenum (black arrow).
- After bowel rest and expectant management, the drainage decreased over 1 month and follow-up contrast injection (Fig. 97.6) demonstrates resolution of the fistulous tract.

Teaching Points

- Persistently high outputs from a drainage catheter should raise the suspicion for a fistulous connection to bowel.

▶ Intermittent drain studies have been shown to decrease the overall catheter dwell time by ensuring optimal position of the catheter in the residual cavity and identifying fistulae. Lastly, intermittent evaluation ensures that the drainage catheter has not eroded into the fistula tract and is providing optimal drainage of the collection.

Management

▶ Depending on output of fistula, measures such as fluid repletion, proximal bowel diversion, or parenteral nutrition may be necessary.

▶ Even in the presence of a persistent fistula, if the output of the catheter is <10 cc, there is no residual abscess cavity, and there is no downstream bowel obstruction, removal of the catheter should be considered.

▶ In some cases, exchange for a straight catheter that can be slowly backed out after every weekly visit may be helpful in allowing the fistula to close.

Further Reading

Gervais DA, Ho CH, O'Neill MJ, et al. Recurrent abdominal and pelvic abscesses: incidence, results of repeated percutaneous drainage, and underlying causes in 956 drainages. *Am J Roentgenol.* 2004; 182:463–466.

History

► Ovarian Cancer and Recurrent Right Pleural Effusion Associated with Dyspnea

What is the best treatment option?

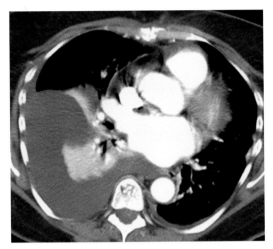

Figure 98.1

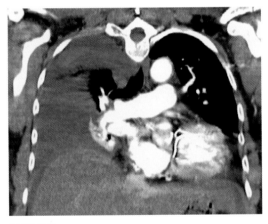

Figure 98.2

Case 98 Tunneled Pleural Catheter

Figure 98.3

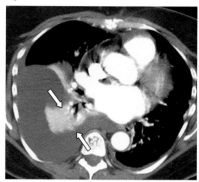

Figure 98.4

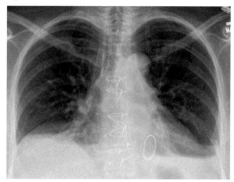

Findings

▶ Axial (Fig. 98.1) and coronal (Fig. 98.2) computed tomography (CT) images show a simple right pleural effusion with associated compressive atelectasis of the right lower lobe (arrows, Fig. 98.3).

▶ After placement of a tunneled pleural catheter, there is decrease in the size of the effusion (Fig. 98.4). Note the catheter is placed at the lung base, in the dependent portion of the hemithorax and courses medially parallel to the spine in the right hemithorax. This course confirms that the catheter is placed posteriorly, in the dependent part of the hemithorax, and not in the fissure, which would provide suboptimal drainage.

Teaching Points

▶ Tunneled pleural catheters are indicated in malignant and refractory pleural effusions. The catheters have a valve to prevent air from entering the pleural space. This is important because negative intrathoracic pressure is generated with every inspiration, and without a valve air could enter and accumulated in the pleural space preventing lung expansion and impeding pleurodesis.

▶ Prior to tunneled pleural catheters, malignant pleural effusions were managed with chest tube placement followed by chemical pleurodesis. This was associated with a prolonged hosptial stay and risks ranging from pain to acute respiratory distress syndrome. In addition, unsuccessful chemical pleurodesis can turn a simple effusion into a complex, multiloculated effusion that is more difficult to treat.

▶ Another advantage of tunneled pleural catheters is that they can be placed as an outpatient procedure and obviate the need for hospitalization. Mechanical pleurodesis following tunneled catheter placement occurs in 50%–60% of patients at a median of 4 weeks after placement and probably results from physiologic inflammation of the visceral pleura caused by the catheter.

▶ In 2013, the FDA approved tunneled pleural catheters include the Pleurx © (Denver Biomedical) and the Aspira© (CR Bard) catheters.

Management

▶ Drainage is performed by the patient or the patient's care partner using specially designed vacuum bottles (Pleurx) or drainage bags (Aspira). Drainage of up to 1 liter every other day is recommended.

▶ When output is <50 cc for three consecutive drainages (over approximately 1 week), repeat chest x-ray is performed. If there is no significant residual, the catheter may be removed.

▶ Alternatively, if there is residual effusion and low output from the catheter, alteplase and/or DNAase can be instilled to disrupt loculations and improve drainage.

Further Reading

Myers R, Michaud G. Tunneled pleural catheters: an update for 2013. *Clin Chest Med.* 2013; 34(1):73–80.

History

▶ A 67-Year-Old Male 2 Weeks Status Post Distal Esophagectomy and Partial Gastrectomy with New Fevers and Leukocytosis

The following studies were performed for workup.

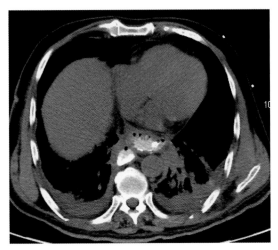

Figure 99.1

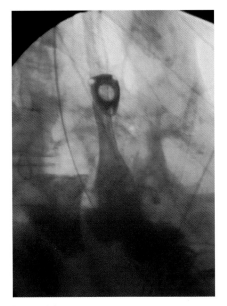

Figure 99.2

Case 99   Anastomotic Leak

Figure 99.3

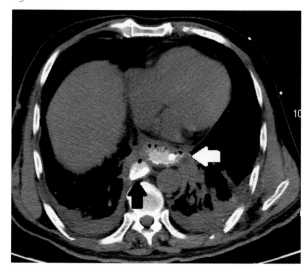

Figure 99.4

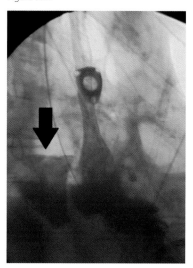

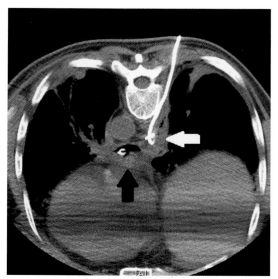

Figure 99.5

Findings

▶ Figure 99.3 is an image at the level of the esophogastric anastamosis from a computed tomography (CT) scan through the chest with oral contrast. An extraluminal collection of contrast is identified (black arrow), just lateral to anastomosis (white arrow).

▶ Esophagram (Fig. 99.4) confirms the diagnosis with extraluminal contrast pooling in the posterior mediastinum (black arrow).

▶ Placement of a drainage catheter within the collection (Fig. 99.5, white arrow) is seen lateral to the esophagus, which is identified by the presence of a nasogastric tube (black arrow).

Teaching Points

▸ Anastamotic leak following esophagectomy is associated with high mortality rate and requires reoperation in up to 24%.

▸ Percutaneous treatment options for esophageal leak include placement of covered esophageal stents or percutaneous drainage.

▸ Care must be taken in placement of these drains to avoid pulmonary parenchyma, esophagus, and major vascular structures.

Management

▸ Catheters should be flushed with 10 mL of saline every 8–12 hours to maintain patency.

▸ Prior to catheter removal, imaging studies are usually performed to confirm the resolution of the leak. Because the leak can be unidirectional (i.e., from the esophagus into the collection but not from the collection back into the esophagus), an esophagram is often performed to confirm closure of the leak rather than an abscessogram.

Further Reading

Arellano RS, Gervais DA, Mueller PR. Computed tomography—guided drainage of mediastinal abscesses: clinical experience with 23 patients. *J Vasc Interv Radiol.* 2011; 22:673–677.

History

► A 36-Year-Old Male Alcoholic with Sudden Severe Chest Pain

Figure 100.1 shows an exam at presentation. Figures 100.2 and 100.3 show interval surgical therapy. You are asked to evaluate Figure 100.3 in this patient with now persistent leukocytosis and fevers.

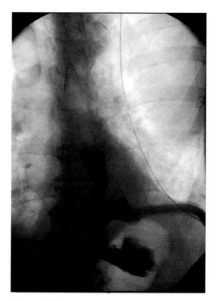

Figure 100.1

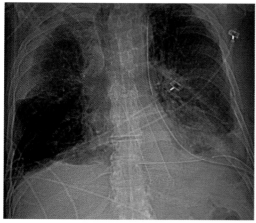

Figure 100.2

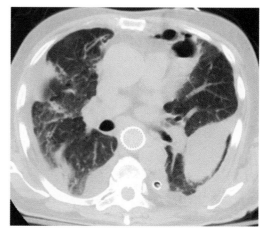

Figure 100.3

Case 100 Esophageal Leak with Persistent locaulated Infected Collection (Empyema)

Figure 100.4

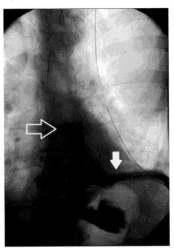

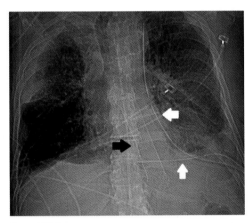

Figure 100.5

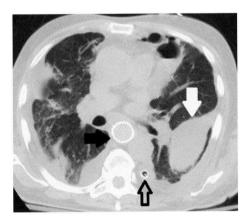

Figure 100.6

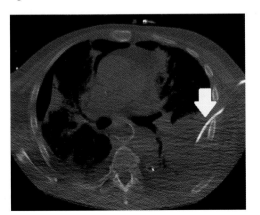

Figure 100.7

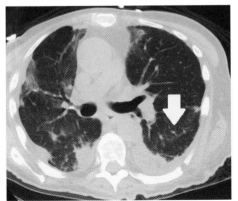

Figure 100.8

Findings

▶ A single contrast esophagram (Fig. 100.4) demonstrates an air-filled esophagus (hollow arrow) with contrast extravasation and drainage into an indwelling basilar chest tube (solid white arrow).

▶ Figure 100.5 shows interval placement of an esophageal stent (black arrow). The left chest tubes remain in place (white arrow).

▶ Computed tomography (CT) image (Fig. 100.6) was obtained for persistent fevers and new leukocytosis. It shows the esophageal stent (solid black arrow) and the basilar chest tubes (hollow black arrow). A loculated fluid collection thought to be the source of persistent infection is identified (white arrow).

▶ Figure 100.7 shows a thoracostomy tube (white arrow), placed under CT guidance secondary to its loculated nature. The drain was kept on suction and injected with alteplase twice during a 2-week course.

▶ One month later a CT (white arrow, Fig. 100.8) shows interval resolution of the loculated collection seen in Figure 100.6.

Teaching Points

▶ Management of complex fluid collections in the thorax is challenging. Etiologies include hemothorax, empyema, and loculated malignant or parapneumonic effusions.

▶ Early treatment is prudent to avoid development of a fibrothorax.

▶ Large-bore tubes (12 French and larger) may be considered in the treatment of complex pleural collections.

Management

▶ Thoracostomy tube may be placed to water seal or low suction. The use intrapleural alteplase (tPA) has been proven to be superior to thoracostomy tube drainage alone.

▶ Addition of intrapleural DNase to alteplase has been shown to be superior to either agent alone in treating patients with complex pleural infections.

▶ Low wall suction may be helpful in re-expansion of ex vacuo pneumothorax, which can be seen after drainage of complex pleural collections due to noncompliance of the underlying lung parenchyma.

Further Reading

Rahman NM, Maskell NA, West A, et al. Intrapleural use of tissue plasminogen activator and DNase in pleural infection. *N Engl J Med.* 2011; 365:518–526.

History

▶ A 56-Year-Old Male with Lymphoma and Jugular Vein Distension, Hypotension, and Tachycardia
What are the treatment options?

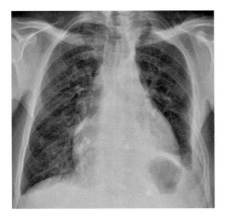

Figure 101.1

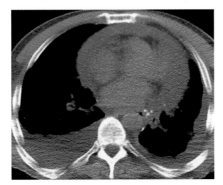

Figure 101.2

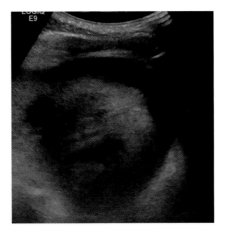

Figure 101.3

Case 101   Pericardial Drain

Figure 101.4

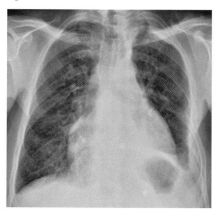

Figure 101.5

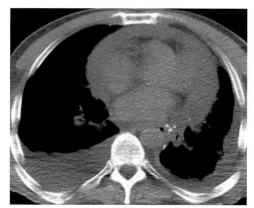

Figure 101.6

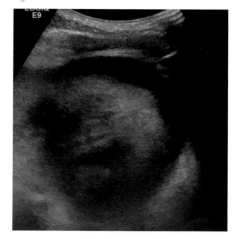

Figure 101.7

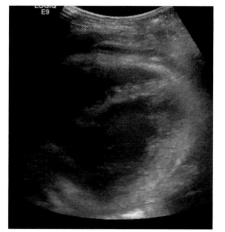

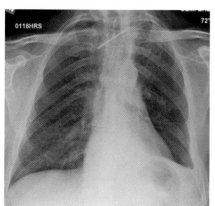

Figure 101.8

Findings

► Anteroposterior radiograph of the chest (Fig. 101.4) shows the characteristic "globoid" or "water bottle" shape of the cardiac sillouhette, which is especially dramatic when compared to a radiograph 1 year earlier (Fig. 101.8).

► Single computed tomography (CT) image and echocardiogram image confirms the presence of a pericardial effusion (Figs. 101.5 and 101.6). On echocardiogram, compression of the right ventricle was seen consitent with tamponade (not shown).

► Immediately after ultrasound guided placement of a percutaneous drain (Fig. 101.7) the effusion has near completely resolved.

Teaching Points

► Common causes of pericardial effusion include malignancy, infection (viral, bacterial, mycobacterial), and connective tissue disease.

► Pericardiac tamponade occurs when the pressure of the intrapericardial fluid compresses the heart. Clinical manifestations include jugular vein distension, muffled heart sounds, hypotension, tachycardia, and dyspnea.

► Echocardiography is the most sensitive imaging tool to confirm the clinical suspicion of tamponade. Findings include engorgement of the vena cavae with reflux into the hepatic veins, paradoxical movement or bowing of the intraventricular septum, and compression of the heart.

► Acute tamponade may occur with relatively little fluid in the pericardium. Chronic pericardial effusion may be significantly larger because the slow accumulation of fluid results in accomodation of the pericardium.

Management

► To determine hemodynamic significance of a pericardial effusion, echocardiography is the best imaging modality because it is portable, inexpensive, and can estimate the fluid volume as well as assess the physiologic consequences of the effusion. Findings on CT suggestive of tamponade include right ventricular wall collapse, and secondary signs of diastolic dysfunction include superior vena cava/inferior vena cava engorgement.

► Pericardial effusion initially causes diastolic dysfunction that can progress to cardiogenic shock with hypotension and decreased cardiac output (decrease pulse pressure).

► Catheter drainage may be definitive treatment. In refractory cases, pericardiodesis with thiotepa or pericardial window may be considered. Percutaneous creation of pericardial window with an angioplasty balloon has been reported.

► Unlike other sites of hemorrhage in which drainage may prevent achieving hemostasis, hemopericardium associated with tamponade needs to be treated with immediate drainage. On rare occasion this complication occurs following biopsy of mediastinal lesions below the superior pericardiac recess, which extends cranially to the the origin of the great vessels.

Further Reading

Palmer SL1, Kelly PD, Schenkel FA, et al. CT-guided tube pericardiostomy: a safe and effective technique in the management of postsurgical pericardial effusion. *Am J Roentgenol.* 2009; 193(4):W314–W320.

Patel N, Rafique AM, Eshaghian S, et al. Retrospective comparison of outcomes, diagnostic value, and complications of percutaneous prolonged drainage versus surgical pericardiotomy of pericardial effusion associated with malignancy. *Am J Cardiol.* 2013; 112(8):1235–1239.

Case 102

History

▸ A 59-Year-Old Male with Hepatitis C Cirrhosis and Liver Mass

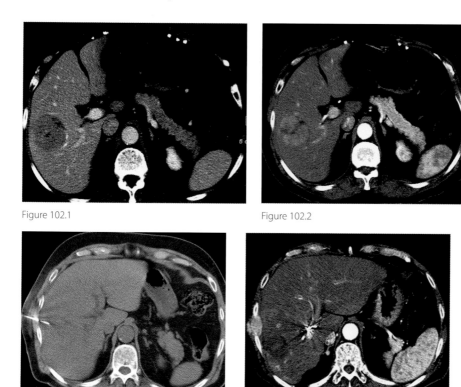

Figure 102.1

Figure 102.2

Figure 102.3

Figure 102.4

Case 102 Needle Tract Seeding Following Biopsy of Hepatocellular Carcinoma

Figure 102.5

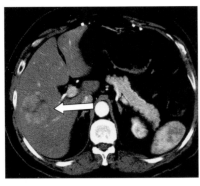

Figure 102.6

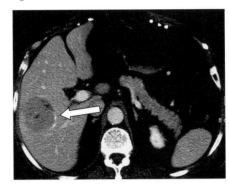

Figure 102.7

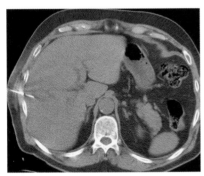

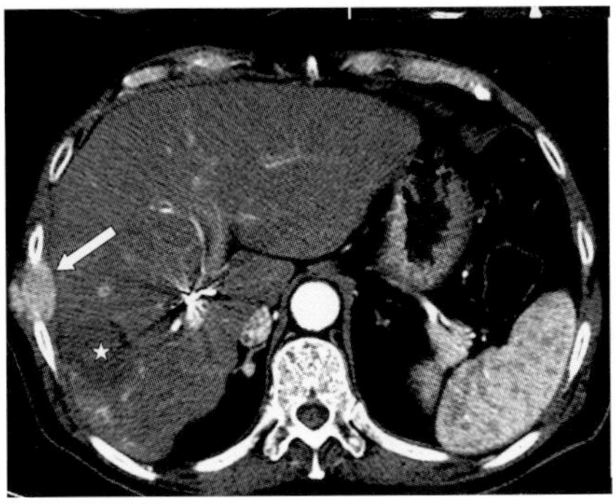

Figure 102.8

Findings

▶ Arterial and portal venous phase computed tomography (CT) (Figs. 102.5 and 102.6, respectively) show an arterially enhancing mass greater than 2 cm in diameter that washes out in portal venous phase imaging.

▶ A coaxial needle is seen in Figure 102.7 targeting the lesion for diagnostic biopsy.

▶ A single image (Fig. 102.8) from an arterial phase CT 18 months later shows an enhancing mass in the abdominal wall corresponding to the site of the previous biopsy (arrow). Notably, the initial hepatic tumor is now smaller and mostly hypovascular (nonviable, star) following intraoperative ablation.

Teaching Points

▶ Diagnosis of hepatocellular carcinoma (HCC) is made based on classic imaging findings—early arterial enhancement with portal venous phase washout on two 3 (or more) phase contrast studies in a lesion >2 cm in size in patients with a known risk factor for HCC. Risk factors for HCC include nonalcoholic steatohepatitis, hepatitis B, and cirrhosis.

▶ Imaging diagnosis of HCC with classic imaging findings in lesions >2 cm is highly specific. Biopsy should be considered only in cases in which imaging findings are indeterminate or for cases in which special studies are required for clinical trials. A Liver Imaging-Reporting and Data System (LI-RADS) classification scheme has been developed to decrease interobserver variability in categorizing liver lesions and to guide treatment, similar to the BI-RADS schema used in breast imaging.

▶ The incidence of tract seeding in HCC in a meta-analysis of 1340 patients was 2.7% but has been reported as high as 5%.

- Tumors related to tract seeding can be seen as soon as 3 months after biopsy or as far out as 4 years.
- The incidence of tract seeding has been hypothesized to be lower with more intervening normal liver parenchyma and use of coaxial biopsy devices. Because of the relatively low incidence, however, neither has been rigorously proven to be of benefit.

Management

- Patients who are potentially transplant candidates should ideally undergo biopsy only after transplant evaluation because tract seeding can convert a patient who is a candidate for curative transplant to a patient with extrahepatic disease precluding transplant.

Further Reading

Silva MA, Hegab B, Hyde C, et al. Needle tract seeding following biopsy of liver lesions in the diagnosis of hepatocellular cancer: a systematic review and meta-analysis. *Gut.* 2008; 57(11):1592–1596.

NCCN Guidelines, Version 2.2013 Hepatocellular carcinoma.

American College of Radiology Quality and safety resources. Liver Imaging-Reporting and Data System. http://www.acr.org/quality-safety/resources/LIRADS. Accessed April 20, 2014.

History

▶ A 63-Year-Old Male Patient, Known to Have Metastatic Lung Cancer, Complaining of 8/10 Low Back Pain Not Responding to Medical Management

What are the procedures being performed?

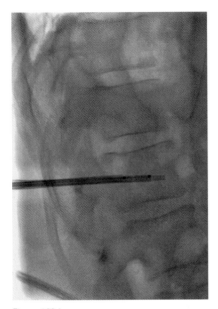

Figure 103.1

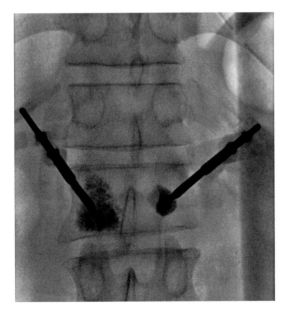

Figure 103.2

Case 103   Left Kyphoplasty and Right Vertebroplasty

Figure 103.3

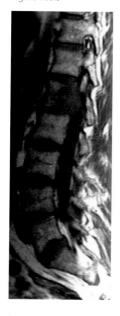

Figure 103.4

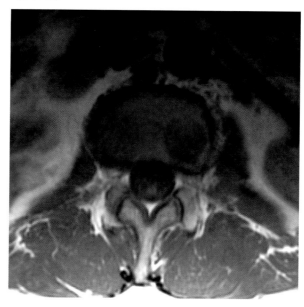

Figure 103.5

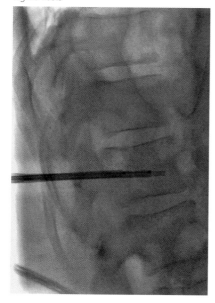

Figure 103.6

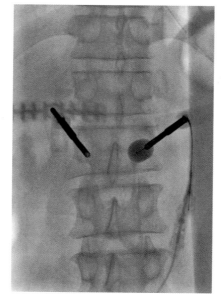

Figure 103.7

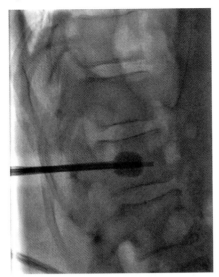

Figure 103.8

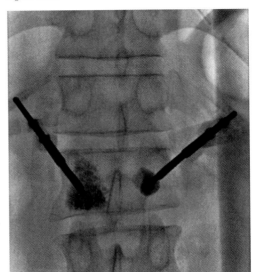

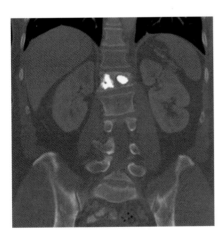

Figure 103.9

Findings

▸ Sagittal and axial T1-weighted magnetic resonance imaging (MRI) (Figs. 103.3, 103.4) show a hypointense metastasis from lung cancer involving the left posterior aspect of the L1 vertebral body.

▸ Lateral image (Fig. 103.5) during positioning of the vertebroplasty needle into the body of L1 via transpedicular approach (Fig. 103.6).

▸ Anteroposterior and lateral projection images during inflation of a balloon on the left side for kyphoplasty, which may restore some of the vertebral body height and reduce the angulation compared to vertebroplasty on the right (Figs. 103.6, 103.7). Anteroposterior image during injection of cement (Fig. 103.8).

▸ Coronal computed tomography (CT) scan (bone window) after the procedure showing radiopaque cement in L1 (Fig. 103.9). No extravasation was seen on axial or sagittal images.

Teaching Points

▸ Percutaneous kyphoplasty and vertebroplasty are safe, minimally invasive procedures performed under imaging guidance for treatment of symptomatic compression fractures secondary to trauma, osteoporosis, malignancy, or painful vertebral hemangiomas.

- There is controversy about the effectiveness of the procedure. Compared to conservative treatment, vertebroplasty and kyphoplasty have been shown to reduce pain both immediately and at 1 year. When compared to a sham procedure, however, two prospective trials published in the *New England Journal of Medicine* found no benefit to vertebroplasty at 6 months.

Management

- Antibiotic prophylaxis is recommended by the Society of Interventional Radiology, typically with 1 g cefazolin.
- Vertebroplasty is performed by advancing a 45-degree beveled-tip needle into the vertebral body under direct image guidance either through the pedicle or via a parapedicular approach. Polymethylmethacrylate (PMMA) cement is injected until cement extends beyond the marrow space. Single-pedicle injection can be used when there is adequate filling of the vertebral body. Otherwise a bipedicular approach is needed.
- Kyphoplasty is a more complex procedure, where a pin is advanced into the vertebral body through the pedicle. A cannula is then advanced over the pin to provide a working channel. A drill inserted through the cannula and is used to create a larger channel in the bone, into which a balloon is inflated to compact the bone and create a cavity to fill with cement.
- It is important to detect any cement leak out of the vertebral body, into either the disc space or a vein in order to avoid complications such as cord compression or pulmonary embolism respectively. When leak is detected, the injection should be stopped and the needle pulled back before resuming cement injection.
- The patient may be moved from the procedure table 20 minutes after confirming adequate solidification of the cement and should be monitored for signs of new radicular pain, spinal compression, and pulmonary embolism.

Acknowledgment

Case courtesy of Bedros Taslakian MD, American University of Beirut Medical Center.

Further Reading

McCall T, Cole C, Dailey A. Vertebroplasty and kyphoplasty: a comparative review of efficacy and adverse events. *Curr Rev Musculoskelet Med.* 2008; 1(1):17–23.

McGraw JK, Cardella J, Barr JD, et al. Society of Interventional Radiology quality improvement guidelines for percutaneous vertebroplasty. *J Vasc Interv Radiol.* 2003; 14:827–831.

Venkatesan AM, Kundu S, Sacks D, et al. Practice guideline for adult antibiotic prophylaxis during vascular and interventional radiology procedures. *J Vasc Interv Radiol.* 2010; 21(11):1611–1630.

Index of Cases

1. Mediport 1
2. Translumbar placement of implantable venous access device 4
3. Left superior vena cava 7
4. Port catheter dislodged from reservoir 10
5. Calcified fibrin sheath 13
6. Lymphangiogram and thoracic duct embolization 16
7. Postbiopsy pneumothorax 19
8. Mediastinal biopsy utilizing separation techniques 22
9. Right coronary artery aneurysm 25
10. Positron emission tomography–guided biopsy 28
11. Adrenal biopsy 31
12. Transcaval pancreatic biopsy 34
13. Autoimmune pancreatitis with biliary tract involvement 37
14. Transjugular liver biopsy 40
15. Renal pseudoaneurysm 43
16. Transperineal magnetic resonance-guided biopsy 46
17. Celiac plexus neurolysis 49
18. Liver biopsy 52
19. Thyroid biopsy 55
20. Placement of fiducial markers to facilitate image-guided radiation therapy 57
21. Hepatocellular carcinoma treated with microwave ablation 60
22. Lung ablation 63
23. Renal cell carcinoma treated with cryoablation 66
24. Cryoablation for pain palliation 69
25. Osteoid osteoma 72
26. Hypertensive crisis during adrenal radiofrequency ablation 75
27. Occluded celiac artery with retrograde flow through gastroduodenal artery 78
28. Liver abscess after embolization 81
29. Transarterial embolization with Y-90 84
30. Hepatic artery aneurysm 87
31. Embolization of renal cell carcinoma bone metastasis 90
32. Bronchial artery embolization 93
33. Pulmonary arteriovenous malformation 96
34. Pelvic congestion syndrome 99
35. Ruptured renal angiomyolipoma 102
36. Liver trauma 105
37. Splenic trauma 108
38. Drainage of abdominal abscess complicated by inferior epigastric artery injury peudoaneurysm 111
39. Upper gastrointestinal bleed 114
40. Lower gastrointestinal bleed 117
41. Juvenile nasal angiofibroma 120
42. Male varicocele embolized with coils and sclerosant 123
43. Partial splenic embolization 126
44. Retrieval of nontarget coil 129
45. Hydronephrosis from obstructing mass failing ureteral stent 132
46. Ureteral-right iliac artery fistula 135
47. Retrograde nephrostomy catheters 138
48. Ureteral stent 141
49. Routine transurethral exchange of ureteral stent 144
50. Occluded ureteral stent 147
51. Uretero-colic fistula treated with urinary diversion and ureteral embolization 150
52. Peritoneovenous shunt placement for chylous ascites 153
53. Percutaneous jejunostomy catheter placement 156
54. Percutaneous cecostomy catheter placement 159
55. Percutaneous pull-through gastrostomy 162
56. Tunneled drainage placement for relief of recurrent ascites 165

57. Internal/external biliary drain   168
58. Intrahepatic biloma   171
59. Primary biliary stent   174
60. Biliary stent complicated by cholecystitis   176
61. Occluded wall stent complicated by cholangitis and cholangitic abscesses   179
62. Varicose veins—greater saphenous vein reflux   182
63. Transjugular intrahepatic portosystemic shunt   185
64. Balloon-occluded retrograde transvenous obliteration of gastric varices   188
65. Adrenal vein sampling   191
66. Superior vena cava syndrome   194
67. Paget Schroetter   197
68. Sclerosis of lymphatic malformation   200
69. May Thurner syndrome   203
70. Inferior vena cava filter placement   206
71. Inferior vena cava filter removal   209
72. Inferior vena cava stent   212
73. Lower-extremity lysis   218
74. Acute pulmonary embolism   224
75. Duplicated inferior vena cava   227
76. Type B aortic dissection and fenestration   230
77. Endoleak   234
78. Traumatic pseudoaneurysm of the carotid artery   237
79. Acute traumatic aortic injury   240
80. Renal artery stenosis   243

81. Femoral artery pseudoaneurysm   246
82. Acute superior mesenteric artery embolism   249
83. Uterine fibroid embolization   252
84. Popliteal entrapment   255
85. Portal vein embolization   257
86. Takayasu's arteritis with ascending aortic aneurysm   260
87. Leriche syndrome   263
88. Thoracic outlet syndrome and subclavian artery aneurysm   266
89. Variant hepatic arterial   268
90. Venous malformation Sclerosis   271
91. Subclavian steal   274
92. Arteriovenous malformation   277
93. Ruptured appendix   280
94. Transgluteal pelvic abscess drainage   282
95. Transrectal aspiration of prostatic abscess   285
96. Sclerosis of traumatic lymphocele   288
97. Small-bowel fistula   291
98. Tunneled pleural catheter   294
99. Anastomotic leak   296
100. Esophageal leak with persistent localuated infected collection (empyema)   299
101. Pericardial drain   302
102. Needle tract seeding following biopsy of hepatocellular carcinoma   305
103. Left kyphoplasty and right vertebroplasty   308

Index

Abdominal abscess
    drainage of, 111–113
    after gastrectomy, 111–113
Abdominal aortic aneurysm
    ascending, 260–262
    endovascular repair of, 234–236
Abdominal pain, 25–27, 37–39, 52–54,
    209–211, 249–251, 280–281
Ablation, 60–77
    cryoablation, 66–68, 69–71
    lung, 63–65
    microwave, 60–62
    radiofrequency, 75–77
Abscesses
    abdominal, 111–113
    cholangitic, 179–181
    after gastrectomy, 111–113
    intrahepatic, 171–173
    liver, 81–83, 180
    pelvic, 282–284
    prostatic, 285–287
Accessory left hepatic artery, 270
Adrenal ademona, 191–193
Adrenal biopsy, 31–33
Adrenal metastasis, 75–77
Adrenal vein sampling, 191–193
AIP. *see* Autoimmune pancreatitis
American Academy of Surgery and Trauma
    Organ Injury scale, 109–110
American Association for the Study of Liver
    Diseases, 53
American Heart Association (AHA)
    suggestions for management of acute PE,
    226
    suggestions for management of DVT,
    222–223
American Society of Diagnostic and
    Interventional Nephrology, 15
American Thyroid Association, 56
AML. *see* Angiomyolipoma

Amplatzer vascular plug, 151, 152
Anastomotic leak, 296–298
Aneurysms. *see also* Pseudoaneurysms
    abdominal aortic, 234–236, 260–262
    hepatic artery, 87–89
    right coronary artery, 25–27
    subclavian artery, 266–267
Angiofibroma, nasal, 120–122
Angiomyolipoma, renal, 102–104
Anterior abdominal collections, 291–293
Anuria, 132–134
Aortic dissection
    type A, 233
    type B, 230–233
Aortic fenestration, 230–233
Aortic injury, traumatic, 240–242
Appendix, ruptured, 280–281
Arterial intervention, 230–279
Arteriovenous malformations
    facial, 277–279
    pulmonary, 96–98
Arteritis, Takayasu's, 260–262
Ascites
    chylous, 153–155
    recurrent after testicular carcinoma
      resection, 153–155
    recurrent in ovarian cancer, 165–167
Aspira© catheter (CR Bard), 294
Atherosclerosis, 263–265
Atrial fibrillation, 249–251
Autoimmune pancreatitis, 37–39
AVMs. *see* Arteriovenous malformations

Back pain
    acute, 230–233
    intractable, 49–51
    low back, 308–311
Balloon fenestration, aortic, 230–233
Balloon-occluded antegrade transvenous
    obliteration, 190

Balloon-occluded retrograde transvenous obliteration, 188–190

BATO. *see* Balloon-occluded antegrade transvenous obliteration

Bile ducts
  high obstruction of, 170, 174–175
  isolation of, 174–175

Biliary catheters, external, 170

Biliary drainage
  indications for, 169, 170
  internal/external placement of, 168–170
  percutaneous, 170

Biliary obstruction
  high, 170, 174–175
  intrahepatic biloma secondary to, 171–173

Biliary stents, 176–178, 179–181

Biloma, intrahepatic, 171–173

Biopsy, 19–59
  adrenal, 31–33
  evaluation for, 25–27
  hepatocellular carcinoma, 305–307
  kidney, 43–45
  liver, 40–42, 52–54
  mediastinal, 22–24, 25–27
  pancreatic, 34–36
  PET-guided, 28–30
  postbiopsy pneumothorax, 19–21
  thyroid, 55–56
  transperineal, 46–48

Bladder cancer, 138–140, 285–287

Bleeding
  gastrointestinal, 114–116, 117–119, 129–131
  nosebleeds, 120–122
  bleeding esophageal varices, 185–187

Blue fingers, 266–267

Bone marrow transplantation, 40–42

Bone metastases
  painful, 69–71
  PET-guided biopsy of, 28–30
  renal cell carcinoma, 90–92

Bowel obstruction
  malignant large-bowel, 159–161
  small-bowel, 156–158

Breast cancer, 28–30, 52–54

Bronchial artery embolization, 93–95

BRTO. *see* Balloon-occluded retrograde transvenous obliteration

Bubble studies, echocardiographic, 96–98

Calf claudication, bilateral, 255–256

Cancer

bladder, 138–140, 285–287
breast, 52–54
cervical, 135–137, 150–152
colon, 63–65, 179–181, 257–259
early-stage carcinoma, 16–18
esophageal, 156–158
gastric, 291–293
hepatocellular carcinoma, 57–59, 60–62, 78–80, 305–307
lung, 69–71, 75–77
ovarian, 141–143, 159–161, 165–167, 224–226, 294–295
pancreatic, 34–36, 49–51, 176–178
renal cell carcinoma, 66–68
testicular carcinoma, 153–155

Cardiac catheterization, 246–248

Cardiac silhouhette, 303, 304

Carotid stents, 237–239

Catecholamine-producing pheochromocytoma, 32, 33

Catheter-directed thrombolysis, 224–226

Catheterization cardiac, 246–248

Catheters
  biliary, 170
  cecostomy, 159–161
  central, 7–9
  cholecystostomy, 178
  dialysis, 13–15
  gastrostomy, 162–164
  implantable venous access devices (IVADs), 1–3, 4–6, 10–12
  internal jugular vein, 3
  jejunostomy, 156–158
  nephrostomy, 138–140
  nephroureteral, 148
  nephroureterostomy, 138–140, 148
  tunneled ascites, 165–167
  tunneled pleural, 294–295

Cecostomy, percutaneous, 159–161

Celiac artery, occluded, 78–80

Celiac plexus neurolysis, 49–51

Central venous catheters, 7–9

Cervical cancer, 135–137, 150–152

Chemical sclerosis, 288–290

Chemotherapy: access for, 4–6
  vascular, 1–3

Chest pain, 260–262, 299–301

Chest tubes, 299–301

Cholangiocarcinoma, 168–170, 174–175

Cholangitic abscesses, 179–181

Cholangitis, 179–181

316

Cholecystectomy, elective laparoscopic, 126–128
Cholecystitis
acute, 176–178
biliary stent placement complicated by, 176–178
Cholecystostomy catheters, 178
Cholelithiasis, symptomatic, 126–128
Chylous ascites, 153–155
Chylous pleural effusion, 16–18
Cirrhosis, 185–187
hepatitis C, 78–80, 305–307
Claudication
calf, 255–256
upper thigh/buttock, 263–265
Colon cancer, 1–3
with liver metastases, 257–259
metastatic, 63–65
post biliary wall stent placement, 179–181
Common carotid artery stents, 239
Congenital heart disease, 7–9
Coronary artery aneurysm, right, 25–27
Craniopharyngioma, 206–208
CR Bard, 294
Creatinine
increasing, 132–134
persistent elevated, 147–149
Crohn's disease, 260–262
Cryoablation
for pain palliation, 69–71
for renal cell carcinoma, 66–68
Cystectomy, 138–140
Cystic hygroma, 202
Cysts, hydatid (echinococcal), 172

Deep vein thrombosis
chronic right lower-extremity, 218–223
iliofemoral, 222, 223
lower-extremity, 227–229
management of, 222–223
Denver Biomedical, 155, 294
Diabetes mellitus, 234–236, 263–265, 285–287
Dialysis catheters, 13–15
Distal esophagectomy, 296–298
Drainage, 280–304
abdominal abscess, 111–113
ascites, 165–167
biliary, 168–170
endoscopic, 169
percutaneous biliary, 170
pericardial, 302–304
small-bowel fistula, 291–293

tunneled, 165–167, 294–295
urinary, 144–146
Drop attacks, 274–276
DVT. see Deep vein thrombosis
Dyspnea, 294–295

Echinococcal (hydatid) cyst, 172
Echocardiographic bubble studies, abnormal, 96–98
Effusions
pericardial, 304
pleural, 16–18, 294–295
Embolism
pulmonary, 206–208, 224–226
superior mesenteric artery, 249–251
Embolization, 78–133, 260–262
bronchial artery, 93–95
gastroduodenal artery, 129–131
hepatic artery, 81–83
hepatocellular carcinoma, 60–62
male varicocele, 123–125
partial splenic, 126–128
for pelvic congestion syndrome, 99–101
portal vein, 257–259
postembolization syndrome, 254
post pancreaticoduodenectomy, 81–83
right radial artery, 90–92
thoracic duct, 16–18
transarterial, with Y-90 particles, 84–86
transcatheter, 125
traumatic liver injury, 106
ureteral, 150–152
uterine fibroid, 252–254
Embolization coils, 131
Embospheres©, 259
Empyema, 299–301
Endograft repair, 240–242
Endoleaks, 234–236
Endoscopic biopsy, pancreatic, 34–36
Endoscopic drainage, 169
Endoscopic stent placement, 176–178
Endovascular aneuruysm repair, 234–236
Enteral feeding access, 156–158
gastrostomy, 162–164
Esophageal cancer, 156–158
Esophageal leak, 298, 299–301
Esophageal stents, 299–301
Esophageal varices, bleeding, 185–187
Esophagectomy
anastomotic leak after, 298
for early-stage carcinoma, 16–18

Facial arteriovenous malformations, 277–279
Facial gunshot wounds, 237–239
Facial swelling, 277–279
Fasciitis, 159–161
Feeding, enteral, 156–158
Femoral artery pseudoaneurysm, 246–248
Fever, 280–281, 296–298
    after biliary stent placement, 176–178, 179–181
    after gastrectomy, 111–113
    after hepatic artery embolization, 81–83
    after right hemicolectomy, 282–284
Fibrin sheaths, calcified, 13–15
Fibroids
    cervical, 254
    intracavitary, 254
    pedunculated subserosal, 254
    uterine fibroid embolization, 252–254
Fiducial markers, 57–59
Filters, inferior vena cava, 206–208, 209–211, 229
Fine-needle aspiration biopsy, pancreatic,
    34–36
Fistulae
    small-bowel, 291–293
    ureteral-right iliac artery, 135–137
    uretero-arterial, 137
    ureterorectal, 150–152
Flank pain
    acute right-sided, 102–104
    right, 147–149

Gastrectomy
    complications of, 111–113
    partial, 291–293, 296–298
Gastric bypass, Roux-en-Y, 114–116
Gastric cancer, 291–293
Gastric pull-up, 156–158
Gastric varices, 188–190
Gastroduodenal artery
    embolization of, 129–131
    retrograde flow through, 78–80
Gastrointestinal/biliary intervention, 153–181
Gastrointestinal bleeding
    embolization of gastroduodenal artery for, 129–131
    lower, 117–119
    upper, 114–116
Gastrorenal shunt, 188–190
Gastrostomy
    pull-through, 162–164
    push-type, 163
Gelfoam slurry, 152
Genitourinary intervention, 135–152
Gooseneck © snares, 148

Greater saphenous vein reflux, 182–184
Gunther Tulip © filter, 211

Haemoglobinuria, paroxysmal nocturnal, 126–128
HCC. see Hepatocellular carcinoma
Heart disease, congenital, 7–9
Hemangioma, hepatic, 171–173
Hematemisis, 188–190
Hematuria, 43–45, 66–68
Hemicolectomy, 282–284
Hemoptysis, massive, 93–95
Hemorrhage. see also Bleeding
    gastrointestinal, 129–131
Hepatic artery
    accessory left, 270
    replaced right, 268–270
    variant anatomy, 268–270
Hepatic artery aneurysm, 87–89
Hepatic artery embolization, 81–83
Hepatic hemangioma, cavernous, 171–173
Hepatic hypertrophy, 257–259
Hepatic venous pressure gradient, elevated,
    40–42
Hepatitis C, 78–80, 185–187, 305–307
Hepatocellular carcinoma, 57–59
    embolized, 60–62
    with hepatitis C cirrhosis, 78–80
    hypervascular segment II, 78–80
    needle tract seeding post biopsy of, 305–307
Hilar cholangiocarcinoma, 170
Huber needle, 3
Hydatid (echinococcal) cyst, 172
Hydronephrosis, 132–134
Hygromas, cystic, 202
Hypertension, 234–236, 302–304
    persistent, 243–245
    renin-dependent, 245
    uncontrolled, 191–193
Hypertensive crisis, 75–77
Hyperthyroidism, 55–56

IFDVT. see Iliofemoral deep venous thrombosis
IGRT. see Image-guided radiation therapy
Ileal conduit, 138–140
Iliac bone metastasis, 28–30
Iliac vein compression syndrome, 205
Iliofemoral deep venous thrombosis, 222, 223
Image-guided liver biopsy, 53
Imaging. see specific modalities
Implantable venous access devices (IVADs),
    1–3, 10–12
    translumbar, 4–6

Inferior epigastric artery pseudoaneurysm, 111–113
Inferior vena cava
    access to, 4–6
    anomalies, 229
    duplicated, 228–229
Inferior vena cava filters
    indications for, 208, 227–229
    indwelling, 212–217
    placement of, 206–208, 209–211
    removal of, 209–211
    suggested locations for, 229
Inferior vena cava stent, 212–217
Inferior venocavagram, 207–208
Injury
    aortic, 240–242
    liver, 106–107
    splenic, 108–110
Internal jugular vein catheters, 3
International Society of the Study of Vascular
    Anomalies Classification System, 202
Intracavitary fibroids, 254
Intrahepatic abscesses, 171–173
Intrahepatic biloma, 171–173
IVADs. see Implantable venous access devices

Jaundice, 37–39
Jejunostomy, 156–158
Jugular vein distenstion, 302–304
Juvenile nasal angiofibroma, 120–122

Kidney biopsy, nontarget, 43–45
Kidney disease, end-stage, 13–15
Kyphoplasty, left, 308–311

Laparoscopic cholecystectomy, elective, 126–128
Large-bowel obstruction, malignant, 159–161
Left upper quadrant pain, 108–110
Leg swelling, chronic bilateral, 212–217
Leriche syndrome, 263–265
Leukocytosis, 296–298
    after biliary stent placement, 176–178,
        179–181
    after gastrectomy, 111–113
    after hepatic artery embolization, 81–83
    after right hemicolectomy, 282–284
    secondary to biliary obstruction, 171–173
Lidocaine, tumescent, 184
Liver abscesses
    causes of, 180
    after embolization post pancreaticoduodenectomy,
        81–83

Liver biopsy, 52–54
    image-guided, 53
    transjugular, 40–42
Liver injury
    grading, 106–107
    traumatic, 106
Liver masses, 52–54, 305–307
Liver metastases
    colon cancer with, 257–259
    neuroendocrine, 268–270
    rectal cancer with, 84–86
Loculated effusions, 294–295
Lower-extremity deep vein thrombosis, acute,
        227–229
Lower-extremity lysis, 218–223
Lower-extremity pain, progressive right, 271–273
Lower-extremity swelling, 203–205
    acute, 218–223
Lower-extremity varicose veins, 182–184,
        203–205
Lower gastrointestinal bleeding, acute, 117–119
Lung ablation, 63–65
Lung biopsy, 19–21
Lung cancer, 4–6
    metastatic, 69–71, 75–77, 308–311
    non-small cell, 22–24
Lymphatic malformations, 200–202
Lymph nodes, mediastinal, 22–24
Lymphoangiography, 16–18
Lymphocele, traumatic, 288–290
Lymphoma, 302–304
    with acute lower-extremity swelling, 218–223
Lysis, lower-extremity, 218–223

Magnetic resonance guidance, 46–48
Male varicocele, 123–125
Malignant ascites, 167
Malignant large-bowel obstruction, 159–161
May Thurnder syndrome, 203–205
Mediastinal biopsy, 22–24
Mediastinal mass, 25–27
Melena, 114–116
Menorrhagia, 252–254
Metastases
    adrenal, 75–77
    bone, 28–30, 69–71, 90–92
    intracranial, 227–229
    liver, 84–86, 257–259, 268–270
Metastatic colon cancer, 63–65
Metastatic lung cancer, 69–71, 75–77, 308–311
Metastatic osseous lesions, 69–71
Metastatic ovarian cancer, 224–226

Microwave ablation, 60–62
Motor vehicle accidents, 288–290
  high-speed, 240–242
  left upper quadrant pain after, 108–110

Nasal angiofibroma, juvenile, 120–122
N-butyl cyanoacrylate (NBCA), 152, 236
Needle tract seeding, 305–307
Nephrolithiasis, 25–27
Nephrostomy
  for hydronephrosis, 132–134
  indications for, 149
Nephrostomy catheters, retrograde, 138–140
Nephroureteral catheters, 148
Nephroureteral stents, 132–134
Nephroureterostomy catheters, 138–140, 148
Neuroendocrine liver metastases, 268–270
Neurolysis, celiac plexus, 49–51
NeuWave microwave probes copyright, 61
Nocturnal haemoglobinuria, paroxysmal, 126–128
Nonalcoholic steatohepatitis, 60–62
Non-small cell lung cancer, 22–24
Nosebleeds, recurrent, 120–122

OK-432 (Pacibinal), 202
Onyx, 236
Option © filter, 211
Osseous lesions, metastatic, 69–71
Osteoid osteoma, 72–74
Ovarian cancer, 141–143, 165–167, 294–295
  metastatic, 224–226
  peritoneal carcinomatosis secondary to,
    159–161

Pacibinal (OK-432), 202
Paget Schroetter syndrome, 197–199
Pain
  abdominal, 25–27, 37–39, 52–54, 209–211,
    249–251, 280–281
  acute back pain, 230–233
  acute right-sided flank, 102–104
  arm, 197–199
  back, 49–51, 230–233, 308–311
  after biliary stent placement, 176–178
  bone metastases, 69–71
  after cardiac catheterization, 246–248
  chest, 260–262, 299–301
  hip, 69–71
  on injection of IVAD, 10–12
  left hip, 72–74
  left upper quadrant, 108–110
  low back, 308–311

lower-extremity, 182–184, 271–273
  pelvic, 285–287
  postprandial, 34–36
  right flank, 147–149
  testicular, 123–125
  upper quadrant, 176–178
Pancreatic biopsy, transcaval, 34–36
Pancreatic cancer, 34–36, 49–51, 176–178
Pancreaticoduodenectomy, 81–83
Pancreatitis, autoimmune, 37–39
Paroxysmal nocturnal haemoglobinuria, 126–128
Partial gastrectomy, 296–298
Pelvic abscesses, 282–284
Pelvic congestion syndrome, 99–101
Pelvic fullness, 99–101
Pelvic masses, 132–134
Pelvic pain, 285–287
Pelvic radiation, 135–137
Percutaneous biliary drainage, 170
Percutaneous biopsy, pancreatic, 34–36
Percutaneous cecostomy, 159–161
Percutaneous kyphoplasty, 308–311
Percutaneous pull-through gastrostomy, 162–164
Percutaneous radiological jejunostomy catheter
    placement, 156–158
Percutaneous vertebroplasty, 308–311
Pericardiac tamponade, 304
Pericardial drain, 302–304
Pericardial effusion, 304
Peripherally inserted central catheter, 7–9
Peritoneal carcinomatosis, 159–161
Peritoneal catheters, tunneled, 167
Peritoneovenous shunts, 153–155
Persistent left superior vena cava, 7–9
Pheochromocytoma, catecholamine-producing,
    32, 33
Pinch-off syndrome, 3, 12
Pleural catheters, tunneled, 294–295
Pleural effusions
  chylous, 16–18
  loculated, 294–295
  right, 294–295
Pleurx© catheter (Denver Biomedical), 294
Pneumothorax, postbiopsy, 19–21
PNH. see Paroxysmal nocturnal haemoglobinuria
Popliteal entrapment, 255–256
Portal vein embolization, 257–259
Positron emission tomography–guided biopsy, 28–30
Postembolization syndrome, 254
Prostatic abscesses, 285–287
Pruritus, intractable, 174–175
Pseudoaneurysms

femoral artery, 246–248
inferior epigastric artery, 111–113
left carotid artery, 237–239
renal artery, 43–45
Pulmonary arteriovenous malformations, 96–98
Pulmonary embolism
acute, 224–226
postoperative, 206–208

Radiation, pelvic, 135–137
Radiation therapy
for cervical cancer, 150–152
image-guided, 57–59
Radiofrequency ablation, adrenal, 75–77
RAS. *see* Renal artery stenosis
Rectal cancer, 84–86
Reflux, greater saphenous vein, 182–184
Renal angiomyolipoma, ruptured, 102–104
Renal artery pseudoaneurysm, 43–45
Renal artery revascularization, 245
Renal artery stenosis, 243–245
Renal cell carcinoma
cryoablation treatment of, 66–68
metastasis to bone, 90–92
Renal disease, end-stage, 13–15
Renin-dependent hypertension, 245
Retention sutures, 159–161
Retroperitoneal sarcoma, 46–48
Right hepatic artery
nontarget coil retrieval from, 129–131
replaced, 268–270
Right iliac artery fistula, 135–137
Right radial artery approach, 90–92
Roux-en-Y gastric bypass, 114–116

"Sandwich" technique, 151, 152
Sarcoma, retroperitoneal, 46–48
Schobinger Scale, 279
Sclerosis
chemical, 288–290
of lymphatic malformation, 200–202
of traumatic lymphocele, 288–290
venous malformation, 271–273
Shortness of breath
acute, 19–21, 224–226
progressive, 96–98
Shunts
gastrorenal, 188–190
peritoneovenous, 153–155
transjugular intrahepatic portosystemic,
185–187
Sickle cell trait, 260–262

"Sling" technique, 211
Small-bowel fistula, 291–293
Small-bowel obstruction, 156–158
Small cell carcinoma, 194–196
Society for Vascular Surgery, 236
Spine augmentaiton, 308–312
Splenic embolization, partial, 126–128
Splenic trauma, 108–110
Squamous cell carcinoma, 162–164
Steal, subclavian, 274–276
Steatohepatitis, nonalcoholic, 60–62
Stents
biliary, 176–178, 179–181
carotid, 237–239
common carotid artery, 239
esophageal, 299–301
inferior vena cava, 212–217
nephroureteral, 132–134
superior vena cava, 195–196
ureteral, 134, 135–137, 141–143, 144–146, 147–149
Stromal tumor seeding, 162–164
Subclavian artery aneurysm, 266–267
Subclavian steal, 274–276
Subclavian vein effort thrombosis, 197–199
Superior mesenteric artery embolism, acute, 249–251
Superior vena cava
calcified fibrin sheath over, 13–15
persistent left, 7–9
Superior vena cava occlusion, 4–6
Superior vena cava stents, 195–196
Superior vena cava syndrome, 194–196
Sutures, retention, 159–161
Swelling
groin, 246–248
lower-extremity, 203–205, 212–217
right neck, 200–202
thigh, 288–290

Tachycardia, 302–304
Takayasu's arteritis
with ascending aortic aneurysm, 260–262
classification of, 262
Testicles, painful swollen, 123–125
Testicular carcinoma, 153–155
Thermal ablation, 68
Thigh swelling, 288–290
Thoracic duct embolization, 16–18
Thoracic outlet syndrome, 266–267
Thrombocytopenia
partial splenic embolization treatment of,
126–128
post bone marrow transplant, 40–42

Thrombolysis, catheter-directed, 224–226
Thyroid biopsy, 55–56
TIPS. *see* Transjugular intrahepatic
    portosystemic shunt
Tract seeding, 305–307
Transarterial embolization, 84–86
Transcatheter embolization, 125
Transjugular intrahepatic portosystemic shunt,
    185–187
Transjugular liver biopsy, 40–42
Translumbar implantable venous access device, 4–6
Transperineal biopsy, MR-guided, 46–48
Transrectal aspiration, 285–287
Trapese © filter, 211
Trauma, splenic, 108–110
Traumatic aortic injury, acute, 240–242
Traumatic liver injury, 106
Traumatic lymphocele, 288–290
Trisegmentectomy, right, 257–259
Tumors, stromal seeding, 162–164
Tunneled ascites catheters, 165–167
Tunneled pleural catheters, 294–295

UFE. *see* Uterine fibroid embolization
Ultrasound guidance
    for IVC access, 4–6
    for liver biopsy, 40–42
    pancreatic biopsy with, 34–36
    for thyroid biopsy, 55–56
Upper gastrointestinal bleeding, 114–116
Upper quadrant pain, left, 108–110
Upper thigh/buttock claudication, 263–265
Ureteral embolization, 150–152

Ureteral obstruction, 141–143
Ureteral-right iliac artery fistula, 135–137
Ureteral stents, 134, 141–143
    complications of, 135–137, 147–149
    indwelling, 135–137
    occluded, 144–146, 147–149
    removal of, 134, 149
    transurethral exchange of, 144–146
Uretero-arterial fistulae, 137
Uretero-enteric anastomotic strictures, bilateral,
    138–140
Ureterorectal fistula, 150–152
Urinary diversion, 150–152
Urinary drainage, 144–146
Urokinase, 152
Uterine fibroid embolization, 252–254

Varicocele, male, 123–125
Varicose veins, lower-extremity, 182–184,
    203–205
Vascular malformations, 202, 271–273
Vascular proliferative neoplasms, 202
Venous access, 1–18
Venous intervention, 182–229
Venous malformation sclerosis, 271–273
Vertebroplasty, right, 308–311

Winslow pathway, 265
Wounds, gunshot, 237–239

Yttrium-90 (Y-90) therapy, 84–86

"Z-type" anatomy, 259